The Potentially Violent Patient and the *Tarasoff* Decision

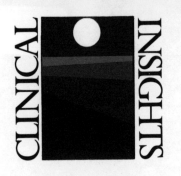

CLINICAL INSIGHTS

The Potentially Violent Patient and the *Tarasoff* Decision in Psychiatric Practice

SCHOOL OF
CALIFORNIA PROFESSIONAL
PSYCHOLOGY
LOS ANGELES

Edited by
JAMES C. BECK, M.D., PH.D.

Assistant Professor of Psychiatry, Harvard Medical School;
Medical Director, Cambridge-Somerville Unit, Metropoli-
tan State Hospital, Waltham, Massachusetts

AMERICAN PSYCHIATRIC PRESS, INC.
Washington, D.C.

© 1985 American Psychiatric Association

Library of Congress Cataloging in Publication Data

Main entry under title:

The potentially violent patient and the *Tarasoff* decision in psychiatric practice.

(Clinical insights)
Includes bibliographies.
1. Psychotherapists—Legal status, laws, etc.—United States. 2. Confidential communications—Physicians—United States. 3. Psychotherapist and patient. I. Beck, James C., 1934- . II. Series. [DNLM: 1. Confidentiality—legislation. 2. Physician-Patient Relations—legislation. 3. Psychotherapy—legislation. 4. Violence—legislation. WM 33 AA1 T17]
KF2910.P75P68   1985   344.73'041   84-28241
                                     347.30441
ISBN 0-88048-075-0 (pbk.)

Printed in the U.S.A.

Contents

Contributors

PAUL S. APPELBAUM, M.D.
Director, Program in Psychiatry and the Law, Massachusetts Mental Health Center; Associate Professor of Psychiatry, Harvard Medical School

JAMES C. BECK, M.D., PH.D.
Assistant Professor of Psychiatry, Harvard Medical School; Medical Director, Cambridge-Somerville Unit, Metropolitan State Hospital, Waltham, Massachusetts

CAROLYN BLITCH, M.A.
Senior Research Associate, Center for Applied Social Research, Northeastern University, Boston

WILLIAM BOWERS, PH.D.
Director, Center for Applied Social Research, Northeastern University, Boston

DAN GIVELBER, J.D.
Professor of Law, Northeastern University School of Law, Boston

MARK J. MILLS, M.D., J.D.
Chief, Psychiatry Service, Veterans Administration Medical Center, Brentwood Division, Los Angeles

Introduction

In the case of *Tarasoff v. Regents of the University of California* (1), the California Supreme Court ruled that the psychotherapist of a potentially violent patient has a duty to protect the intended victim from the patient's threatened violence. This decision has generated considerable concern among psychiatrists and other mental health professionals, many of whom remain convinced that the *Tarasoff* doctrine is inimical to the practice of their profession. At the same time, surveys show that many psychotherapists, including psychiatrists, are ignorant or misinformed about what a *Tarasoff* standard of professional conduct requires of them. Furthermore, because legal doctrine is developing case by case and state by state, experts as well as practicing clinicians have difficulty maintaining an accurate assessment of the legal ground rules under which they practice.

Patients whom the therapist fears may be violent are always difficult to treat. The difficulties are now compounded by the uncertainties associated with the *Tarasoff* decision. Because most therapists treat relatively few such patients, they lack the extensive clinical experience that provides a basis for confidence in difficult clinical situations. For some therapists, the difficulty of treating potentially violent patients may be increased because their attention is divided between their concern for the clinical issues and their concerns about their legal obligations. More psychiatrists consult the American Psychiatric Association (APA) legal consultation service about the *Tarasoff* duty than about any other issue.

The purpose of this monograph is to present, primarily for psychiatrists and other psychotherapists, a review of the relationship between the *Tarasoff* doctrine and clinical practice. Since the first *Tarasoff* decision in 1974, there has been a developing body of case law, and of systematic empirical investigation, concerning how the *Tarasoff* duty affects clinical practice. Some clear, concrete, practical implications for clinical practice have emerged from this work.

This monograph is organized into two major divisions. The first four chapters are devoted primarily to reporting relevant facts: legal cases the Courts have decided, and clinical cases and research data we have collected. Chapter One presents a review of the original *Tarasoff* case, including the clinical facts, the two California Supreme Court decisions, and the role of the APA in the case. Chapter Two provides a review of the relevant legal cases in which the *Tarasoff* doctrine has evolved since 1974. The central legal issue, as well as the variations in how individual Courts have dealt with it, emerges from this historical review. Chapter Three reports on the results of a national survey of psychiatrists and other psychotherapists concerning their knowledge of *Tarasoff*, their attitudes toward it, and how their clinical practice has changed under *Tarasoff*. Chapter Four describes clinical experience with *Tarasoff* cases, and draws some clinical inferences from them.

The second major portion of the monograph is devoted to an analysis of the clinical implications of the facts as presented in the first four chapters. Chapter Five explains why psychiatrists' predictions of violence are necessarily inaccurate, and why this inaccuracy has nothing to do with clinical skills or acumen. The implications of this explanation for improving clinical practice with potentially violent patients, and for avoiding legal liability, are also presented. Chapters Six and Seven are devoted to the implications of *Tarasoff* for clinical practice. Chapter Six contains a theoretical analysis of the *Tarasoff* duty, which provides a framework for understanding what is required of the clinician. Chapter Seven builds on that framework to describe explicitly how the clinician should conduct himself so as to fulfill the *Tarasoff* duty. The clinician who wants to know what to do can go directly to this chapter. Chapter Eight summarizes the most important observations and analyses presented in the first seven chapters, and draws conclusions based on them.

The analyses presented by the authors of the several chapters are theirs alone. None of our work represents the viewpoint, official or unofficial, of the American Psychiatric Association, and it should not be taken as such. The authors do not always agree. The editor has encouraged each author to write his own chapter. Suggested editorial changes were designed to insure continuity, not agreement.

James C. Beck, M.D., Ph.D

References

1. *Tarasoff v. Regents of the University of California*, 17 Cal. 3d 425, 551 P.2d 334 (1976)

1

The *Tarasoff* Case

Mark J. Mills, J.D., M.D.
James C. Beck, M.D., Ph.D.

1

The *Tarasoff* Case

Prosenjit Poddar, Indian by nationality and untouchable by caste, was a graduate student at the University of California at Berkeley when he met Tatiana Tarasoff at a folk dance in the autumn of 1968 (1). They saw each other weekly at social events, and on New Year's Eve he kissed her. He thought the relationship was serious; she told him it was not. Thereafter, he became withdrawn, neglected his work, and often cried. He had tape recorded several conversations with Tatiana, and spent hours dissecting these conversations with his roommate. In the summer of 1969, Ms. Tarasoff went to South America. Poddar entered outpatient psychotherapy at the Cowell Memorial Hospital of the University of California.

Contrary to his usual practice, the psychiatrist who evaluated Poddar at Cowell told him during the first interview that Poddar was quite disturbed. The psychiatrist, who was a member of the inpatient staff, decided that Poddar did not require hospitalization. He prescribed a neuroleptic, and referred Poddar to a psychologist on the outpatient staff for weekly psychotherapy. During this therapy, on August 18 (2), Poddar expressed fantasies of harming, or perhaps even killing, Ms. Tarasoff. The therapist also learned, from a friend of the patient, that the patient planned to purchase a gun. Deeply concerned about Poddar's potential for violence, the

2

therapist consulted his supervising psychiatrist and the psychiatrist who had initially evaluated Poddar. Having decided that Poddar required hospitalization, the therapist telephoned and then wrote to the campus police on August 20 (2), citing the fact that his illness and dangerousness fit California's civil commitment criteria. They requested police aid in committing him.

At this time, California's then novel civil commitment statute, the Lanterman–Petris–Short Act, had been in effect only two months. Thus, none of the key parties—the psychiatrists, the psychologist, or the campus police—were experienced with the new civil commitment procedure. They all made mistakes. Under the law, the city police, not the university police, should have been contacted, and they should have transported Poddar to a county facility for an emergency psychiatric evaluation. In fact, the campus police went to Poddar's apartment, where they questioned him about his intended behavior. Poddar denied any violent intentions, and the police left after warning him to stay away from Ms. Tarasoff. The mental health professionals took no further action to detain Poddar. Poddar dropped out of treatment some time after August 18.

Poddar subsequently moved in with Ms. Tarasoff's brother. In October 1969, after Ms. Tarasoff had returned from South America, Poddar went to her home. She was out, and her mother asked him to leave. Returning later with a pellet gun and a butcher knife, Poddar found Ms. Tarasoff home alone. She refused to talk with him and began to scream. He shot her with the pellet gun, and she ran from the house. He followed her and stabbed her to death.

Following her death, the state charged Poddar with first degree murder (3). Subsequently, the Tarasoffs sued the University, including both the campus police and the student health service psychotherapists. This civil suit became the *Tarasoff* case (1). The Tarasoffs alleged that the police had been negligent in not detaining Poddar, and that the psychotherapists had been negligent in not warning Ms. Tarasoff of Poddar's threats and in not confining him. The defendants—the University of California— demurred: that is, they argued that even if the plaintiff's allegations were true, there was no legal duty on the part of either the police or the psychotherapists to protect or to warn. Accepting this argument, the court dismissed the Tarasoff's complaint on the grounds that it failed to state a cause of action (2). The Tarasoffs appealed (1).

In 1974, the California Supreme Court held that on the facts alleged in the complaint, the psychotherapist had a duty to warn. "When a doctor or a psychotherapist, in the exercise of his professional skill and knowledge, determines, or should determine, that a warning is essential to avert danger arising from the medical or psychological condition of his patient, he incurs a legal obligation to give that warning (1, p. 914). On the issue of the psychotherapists' failure to confine Poddar, the Court found the defendants immune. The Court also found that the University police were immune from liability, because California's civil commitment statute mandates broad immunity to those releasing civil commitment detainees.

At this point the American Psychiatric Association (APA), in collaboration with other professional organizations, filed an *amicus curiae* brief asking the Court to rehear the appeal (4). The amici were concerned that requiring therapists to warn potential victims would lead to frequent breaches of the patient's right to confidentiality. They argued that, given the rarity of violence, many predictions would necessarily be falsely positive. Therefore, most of these breaches would serve no purpose other than to create anxiety in the potential victim, and would, coincidentally, undermine the patient's confidence in the therapist and in the therapeutic process. The brief appeared to assume a fact situation similar to that in the *Tarasoff* case, one in which the therapist would take action to protect the victim without first discussing this decision with the patient. The brief stated, "When a psychotherapist is compelled to, and does draw the conclusion that his patient may become violent, the therapist's own actions may well betray this judgment to the patient" (4, p. 24).

Not only were concerns raised about breaches of confidentiality in the event of potential danger, but some psychotherapists believed they would be obliged to alert patients routinely about the duty to warn (5). They considered the effect of telling a patient at the outset of psychotherapy that certain things the patient might say could trigger a warning to third parties. They worried about the "chilling effect" such a warning would have in preventing the patient from disclosing affect-laden fantasies, a process essential to accomplishing the work of psychotherapy (6).

Because of the importance of these issues and the continuing concern expressed by the APA and others, the California Supreme Court agreed to rehear the case, and in 1976 issued a second opinion (7). The Court again held that a psychotherapist has a duty to the potential victim, but defined that duty more broadly and with more latitude for professional judgment by the therapist. The Court said, "When a therapist determines or pursuant to the standard of his profession should determine, that his patient presents a serious danger of violence to another, he incurs an obligation to use reasonable care to protect the intended victim against such danger. The discharge of this duty may require the therapist to take one or more of various steps depending upon the nature of the case. Thus it may call for him to warn the intended victim or others likely to apprise the intended victim of danger, to notify the police, or take whatever steps are reasonably necessary under the circumstances" (7, p. 346). The second opinion thus modified the duty to warn as defined in in the first *Tarasoff* opinion, making it in effect a duty to protect.

The Court's opinion was not unanimous: four of seven judges concurred. Judge Mosk agreed that there was a cause of action because defendants did predict violence and failed to warn. He doubted that the facts would support a finding of negligence because the defendants had notified the police. However, on the broader question of holding psychotherapists liable for failing to predict violence he dissented, saying, "I cannot concur, however, in the majority's rule that a therapist may be held liable for failing to predict his patient's tendency to violence if other practitioners, pursuant to the 'standards of the profession,' would have done so. The question is, what standards? . . . psychiatrist predictions of violence are inherently unreliable" (7, p. 354). In a separate dissent, Judge Clark agreed with the amici that the new duty would not increase public safety. He said, "the majority fails to recognize that . . . overwhelming policy considerations mandate against sacrificing fundamental patient interests without gaining a corresponding increase in public benefit" (7, p. 355).

Judge Tobriner, writing for the majority, said that the basis for the therapist's duty to protect was the "special relationship" existing between the therapist and patient, but failed to state the basis for the opinion that such a special relationship exists. Nor did the opinion specify who is subject to this duty. The case involved a psychologist and a psychiatrist, but what about social workers, nurse-therapists, or counselors? The opinion did not spell out the steps necessary to discharge the duty of protection. Most important, it left unstated how the therapist is to know when he should determine or how he should try to determine that his patient presents a danger of violence to another.

Because of its ambiguity, the Court's second ruling caused even more anxiety than the first. There were frequent discussions among psychotherapists about how the new duty could be discharged (5); for example, if the psychotherapist attempts to warn by telephone and there is no answer, is a registered letter sufficient, or should one call the police?

Viewing the California Court as a judicial bellwether, some jurists predicted that the *Tarasoff* opinion would be the first of many that would impose a similar duty on psychotherapists in other jurisdictions (8). Subsequent cases have partially confirmed these predictions. Courts in an increasing number of states have held that psychotherapists have a duty to protect possible victims of a patient's potentially violent behavior. The specifics of the duty vary from state to state; for example, whether the therapist has a duty to all potential victims or only to named potential victims, whether particular actions satisfy the duty or whether others are required. The next chapter summarizes this recent case law.

References

1. *Tarasoff v. Regents of the University of California*, 118 Cal. Rptr. 129, 529 P.2d 553 (1974)

2. *Tarasoff v. Regents of the University of California*, 108 Cal. Rptr. 878 (1973)

3. *People v. Poddar*, 103 Cal. Rptr.84 (1972)

4. Brief in support of Respondent's petition for Rehearing *Tarasoff v. Regents of University of California*, 17 Cal. 3d 425, 551 P2d 334, 131 Cal. Rptr.14 (1976)

5. Wise TP: Where the public peril begins: a survey of psychotherapists to determine the effects of *Tarasoff*. Stanford Law Review 31:165–190, 1978

6. Stone A: The Tarasoff decisions: suing psychotherapists to safeguard society. Harvard Law Review 90:358–370, 1976

7. *Tarasoff v. Regents of the University of California*, 17 Cal. 3d 425, 551 P.2d 334 (1976)

8. Appelbaum PS: The expansion of liability for patients' violent acts. Hosp Community Psychiatry 35:13-14, 1984

2

The Psychotherapist and the Violent Patient: Recent Case Law

James C. Beck, M.D., Ph.D.

2

The Psychotherapist and the Violent Patient: Recent Case Law

To understand the recent legal history of the *Tarasoff* doctrine and its application to clinical work, the clinician needs some introduction to the legal issues. Many clinicians resent the increasing extent to which clinical work appears to be influenced by legal constraints. Knowledge of the facts of some recent Court cases may give the reader an increased sense that the Courts are attempting to deal constructively with difficult issues concerning both psychiatry and the law.

In all the cases to be presented, the Court considers two types of questions: questions of law and questions of fact. In all of these cases, the primary question of law is whether the defendant owed a *Tarasoff* duty to the plaintiff. If there was such a duty, the factual questions are: did the defendant breach this duty; was the plaintiff damaged; and did the defendant's conduct "proximately" cause the plaintiff's damages? If the answer to all four of these questions is affirmative, the plaintiff may recover for the defendant's negligence.

The first question, whether a legal duty exists, typically begins with a discussion of the *Tarasoff* duty and whether it applies in the Court's jurisdiction. In addition to *Tarasoff*, many Courts consider paragraph 315 of the *Second Restatement of Torts*, a basic legal treatise in this field (1). Paragraph 315 states an exception to the general rule of Tort law that under ordinary circumstances one person does not have any duty to act so as to prevent harm from befalling some other person. If I see a man drowning, I am under no legal obligation to prevent or try to prevent him from drowning. If I see a blind woman about to walk in front of a truck, I have no legal obligation to shout, "Stop." The rule governing the exception to this general rule is set out in paragraph 315, which states:

> There is no duty so to control the conduct of a third person as to prevent him from causing physical harm to another unless:
> *a.* a special relation exists between the actor and the third person which imposes a duty upon the actor to control the third person's conduct; or
> *b.* a special relation exists between the actor and the other which gives to the other a right to protection (1).

To a non-lawyer, this language is confusing. The restatement involves three people. A third person, whom the statement mentions first, is the one who actually does the damage. The next person mentioned is the actor, who is the defendant, the one who should or should not have done something different from what he or she did. Finally, the last person mentioned is the other, and this is the person injured, who is typically the plaintiff.

In the typical suit involving a psychiatrist whose patient injures someone else, paragraph 315 might be restated to read:

> A psychiatrist (or other psychotherapist) has no duty so to control the conduct of a patient as to prevent him from causing physical harm to another unless:
> *a.* a special relation exists between the psychiatrist and the patient which imposes a duty upon the psychiatrist to control the patient's conduct; or
> *b.* a special relation exists between the psychiatrist and the victim which gives the victim a right to protection.

Restated in terms describing the patient-therapist relationship, the issue is one that many psychiatrists have repeatedly grappled with, and to which they find no easy answers. The law finds no easy answers, either.

After the Court delineates the legal duty in each of the cases to be presented, it addresses the second question: whether the facts of th case warrant a finding that the defendant was negligent. In determining this issue, the Courts often consider whether or not the violence that occurred was foreseeable. Prosser, the author of the classic text on torts, says, "The test as respects foreseeability is not the balance of probability, but the existence, in the situation in hand, of some real likelihood of some damage and the likelihood is of such appreciable weight and moment as to induce, or which reasonably should induce, action to avoid it on the part of a person of reasonably prudent mind" (2, p. 148). The Courts tend to conclude that a danger is foreseeable if the patient threatened a specific, identifiable victim. Where the threat is more general or nonspecific, opinions divide on whether or not there is a duty to protect.

In each case summarized below, the Court makes a finding concerning the *Tarasoff* duty. The cases are grouped according to their relationship to the *Tarasoff* duty: the *Tarasoff* duty was present; the duty was present and its scope was enlarged; the duty was present, but not in the instant case; the duty was denied.

Some of the cases to be presented involve patients in outpatient psychotherapy. Of these, some were previously hospitalized, and others were not. Other cases involve former inpatients who were discharged but received no outpatient treatment.

The cases involving only inpatient treatment without any aftercare have been less affected by the *Tarasoff* decision than have been the outpatient cases. Prior to *Tarasoff*, psychiatrists and institutions had a duty to use reasonable care to protect society from violent acts by institutionalized patients. Typically, psychiatrists were found negligent in suits based on violence committed by former inpatients only if the psychiatrists departed from generally accepted standards of care. Since *Tarasoff*, these suits include a new cause of action, namely that the defendant psychiatrist or institution failed to protect the potential victim. As a practical matter, these suits appear to be little different from those brought under the older theories of negligence. Typically, the psychiatrist is not found negligent unless there is evidence of a departure from accepted standards of care. Because they appear to create few new concerns for psychiatrists, most of these cases will be summarized only briefly.

THE *TARASOFF* DUTY ADOPTED

In *McIntosh v. Milano* (3), New Jersey Superior Court, 1979, Mrs. McIntosh brought a wrongful death action against a psychiatrist after one of his patients murdered her daughter. The patient in question was a 17-year-old male at the time of the murder, and the victim was a 20-year-old woman with whom he apparently had a sexual relationship. He had begun psychotherapy two years previously. He was diagnosed as having a drug problem and a schizoid character. In therapy, he had expressed fantasies of being afraid of others, being a hero or an important villain, and using a knife to intimidate others. He carried a knife in order to be able to show it to people who tried to intimidate him, and he brought it to a therapy session and showed it to his psychiatrist. The patient told the therapist that he had fired a BB gun at a car in which he thought the victim was riding with her boyfriend. However, the psychiatrist denied that the patient had ever expressed any feeling of violence toward the victim or made any threats to kill or hurt her.

On the day of the murder the patient had fallen off his bicycle and hurt his face. He stole a prescription pad from his psychiatrist and wrote a prescription for 30 Seconal tablets. A suspicious pharmacist checked with the psychiatrist, and then refused to fill it. The patient then took a gun from his home and waited for the victim to visit her parents, persuaded her to go with him to a local park, and fatally shot her in the back. He was convicted of first degree murder, but the conviction was reversed on appeal because of "improper and prejudicial remarks during the trial by the assistant prosecutor." The patient later entered a plea of *non vult* to the murder charge, equivalent to a plea of guilty.

The plaintiff claimed that the psychiatrist had a duty to protect the victim, and that there was ample evidence of the patient's dangerousness. The defendant moved for summary judgment on the legal grounds that he had no duty to the victim, that the *Tarasoff* case had been wrongly decided, that the duty was unworkable, that it would interfere with psychotherapy by breaching confidentiality, that it would deter therapists from treating violent patients, and that it would lead to an increase in commitments—many of the same arguments that the American Psychiatric Association (APA) had made in its *amicus curiae* brief to the California Supreme Court.

The Court held that *Tarasoff* did apply, and that the duty to protect was based on the patient-therapist relationship. The Court also found a more general duty to protect society, analogous to the physician's duty to warn others of carriers of contagious disease. The Court further concluded that confidentiality was not an overriding concern; nor was it impressed with the defendant's other arguments.

When the case was tried, the defendant was found not to have violated his duty.

In *Davis v. Lhim* (4), Michigan Wayne County Circuit Court, 1981, the defendant psychiatrist treated the patient in a state hospital during three voluntary admissions between July and September, 1975. The patient carried diagnoses of schizophrenia, heroin addiction, and alcoholism. On September 3, the patient asked for and received a voluntary discharge. According to a social worker's notes, the patient was told he could not use the hospital as "a motel" to get away from problems at home.

At the time of his release, the patient's mother, with whom he customarily lived in Detroit, was visiting relatives in Alabama, so the patient stayed with an aunt. When he became difficult to manage she took him to his mother. Two months after his discharge, he began firing a shotgun in the house where his mother was staying. His mother tried to talk him out of shooting again, then attempted to restrain him. In the struggle, he fired several more shots, one of which killed his mother.

A jury awarded $500,000 to the victim's estate. The psychiatrist appealed. He argued that the presence of a gun in the household and the attempt to disarm the son were unforeseeable intervening causes of death.

The Appeals Court held that *Tarasoff* was applicable in Michigan, but that it applied only to victims readily identifiable as foreseeably endangered, not to the public at large. The Court concluded that the mother was a foreseeable victim, citing the facts that in 1973 a hospital record noted that the patient "paces the floor and acts strangely and threatens his mother for money," that he had no money on admission, and that as a known drug and alcohol dependent person he would need money.

The Court held that the jury could have found that the defendant had a duty to use reasonable care to protect the patient's mother, and that his negligence was the proximate cause of her death. The Court said it was well known that many persons keep handguns, and that a person threatened with a gun will attempt to disarm the assailant. Based on this reasoning, the Court upheld the jury verdict and the award of $500,000.

Comment: On the facts presented, this decision seems questionable. There was no allegation that the defendant failed to conform to usual professional standards in his diagnosis and treatment of this patient. The fact that the shooting occurred two months after discharge and in a distant city raised questions about how foreseeable this was. Why did the aunt choose to take him to Alabama rather than to a psychiatric facility if he was difficult to manage? The social worker's note raises the possibility that the hospital gave the patient and his family the message that he was using the hospital inappropriately. That message would certainly make it more difficult for the family to turn to the mental health system for help. In that case, one could argue that the family should be compensated.

In *Chrite v. U.S.* (5), U.S. District Court, Michigan, 1983, the Veterans Administration (V.A.) discharged a mental patient, who killed his mother-in-law six months later. On the day he was committed to the hospital, the patient wrote a note saying he was wanted for "murder mother-in-law." The plaintiff claimed that the defendant was negligent in releasing the patient and in not warning the mother-in-law.

On a motion by the defendant for summary judgment, the Court held that the defendant was not liable for releasing the patient. Citing *Davis*, the Court held that the *Tarasoff* duty did apply, so that the defendant could be liable for failing to warn the mother-in-law. The question of whether the defendant is liable has yet to be litigated.

In *Jablonski v. U.S.* (6), U.S. Court of Appeals for the Ninth Circuit, 1983, a child, Meghan Jablonski, sued the V.A. for the wrongful death of her mother. The mother was murdered by a man with whom she had been living. The murderer was a V.A. patient.

On July 7, 1978, the veteran attacked the victim's mother, Meghan's grandmother, with a sharp object and apparently attempted to rape her. She had also received malicious and obscene telephone calls that the police believed came from him. She did not file charges, but discussed with the police the possibility of his receiving psychiatric treatment. He agreed to voluntary treatment, and the police immediately called the V.A. hospital. Because the doctor assigned to treat the patient was not available, the police spoke with the chief of psychiatry. The policeman told the chief about the patient's past criminal record, the recent obscene phone calls, and his own belief that the veteran needed hospitalization. The chief said he would transmit this information to the admitting doctor, but failed to do so.

On Monday, July 10, the victim drove the veteran to the hospital where he saw the psychiatrist. The psychiatrist learned that the patient had served a five year prison term for raping his wife, and that he had attempted to rape Meghan's grandmother four days earlier. The patient said that he had undergone psychiatric treatment, but refused to say where. The psychiatrist diagnosed the patient as a potentially dangerous antisocial personality. The patient was offered voluntary hospitalization, but refused. The psychiatrist thought the patient did not meet standards for involuntary commitment, and offered him an appointment for two weeks hence. Privately, the victim told the psychiatrist that she felt insecure around the patient and was concerned about his unusual behavior. The doctor recommended that she leave him, at least temporarily, but she refused, saying she loved him.

The defendants made no attempt to obtain the patient's past medical history. At trial, an expert testified that local V.A. records could have been obtained by telephone without the patient's permission. If obtained, his records would have revealed a hospitalization in the army in 1968. These records showed that the patient had a history of homicidal ideation toward his wife, had made numerous attempts to kill her, and had probably suffered a psychotic break; that there was a distinct possibility of future violence, and a family history in which his father frequently beat his mother. The diagnosis was undifferentiated schizophrenia.

On July 11 or 12, the victim's mother telephoned the psychiatrist and complained that the next appointment was too far in the future. The psychiatrist persuaded her not to call the police, and agreed to see the patient on Friday, July 14. On July 12, the victim and her daughter moved out of the patient's apartment. On July 14, the patient met with the psychiatrist and his supervisor. Both doctors thought this was an emergency, and that he was dangerous, but not committable. They gave him a prescription for diazepam and scheduled him for more tests.

During this appointment the victim told a third psychiatrist that she was afraid of the patient. This psychiatrist advised her to stay away from him if she was afraid of him. On Sunday, July 16, the victim went back to the apartment, apparently to pick up some diapers, and the patient murdered her.

The District Court found the hospital liable because it failed to record and communicate the warning from the police, because it failed to secure the patient's prior records, and because it failed to warn the victim. These failures proximately caused the victim's death.

On appeal, the government argued that it owed no duty to the victim, first, because no special relationship existed between the patient and the doctors, and, second, because she was not a foreseeable victim. Next, it argued that even if it had such a duty, it had discharged it. Finally, the government argued that the victim received adequate warning from a number of sources. Finding that the District Court's conclusions were not clearly erroneous, the Court of Appeals affirmed the judgment for the plaintiff.

Comment: This is the only case to date in which negligence for breach of a *Tarasoff* duty has been found when the patient was only a psychotherapy patient, and not involved in some more intensive treatment.

Acknowledging that there were shortcomings in the patient's care, it is unclear how the defendants could have done anything that would have protected this victim further. Even if they had known the past medical history, it is questionable whether the patient was committable under California statute, which requires mental illness as one necessary condition for commitment. The patient's only diagnosis was antisocial personality, an Axis Two personality disorder. Typically, at least in San Diego, a person with antisocial personality would not be considered committable (Jay Flocks, M.D., personal communication).

That the patient had, in 1968, been given a diagnosis of schizophrenia tells us little about whether he met current criteria for schizophrenia, especially since the record noted only a question of a psychotic episode. Furthermore, there is no suggestion that the patient was currently psychotic. If the defendants could not commit this patient, what else could they have done for this victim? They warned her, and so did a number of other people, but she persisted in putting herself into a situation that she knew or should have known was highly dangerous.

It is unclear why the psychiatrist advised the victim's mother not to call the police. If she had been willing to make a criminal complaint, the patient could possibly have been incarcerated either in jail or in a hospital, and been evaluated forensically. This strategy is more appropriate for dealing with dangerous antisocial persons who have committed crimes than the strategy that was chosen. Whether the defendant's choice was grounds for malpractice is another question.

In *MacDonald v. Clinger* (7), New York Supreme Court, Appellate Division, 1982, a patient brought action against his psychiatrist for damages for disclosing confidential information to the patient's wife. The psychiatrist moved to dismiss, and this suit was denied. The psychiatrist appealed the denial.

The published facts are sparse. The court held that a *Tarasoff* duty applies in New York. It said that, "disclosure of confidential information by psychiatrist to patient's spouse will be justified whenever there is danger to patient, spouse or another person; otherwise, information should not be disclosed without authorization" (7, p. 802). The court affirmed the denial.

THE *TARASOFF* DUTY ENLARGED

In *Lipari v. Sears, Roebuck and U.S.* (8), U.S. District Court, Nebraska, 1980, the plaintiff alleged that Sears, Roebuck and the V.A. had been negligent. The injuries were caused by a patient of the V.A. who had been hospitalized and discharged to day treatment, from which he apparently dropped out. In September 1977 he bought a shotgun at Sears. On September 23, he resumed day care, and on October 17 he dropped out against medical advice. On November 26, he fired his shotgun in a crowded Omaha nightclub, killing Mr. Lipari and wounding his wife.

Mrs. Lipari brought suit against Sears, Roebuck for selling the patient the gun, claiming the store should have known he was dangerous. Sears, in turn, filed a claim against the V.A. on the grounds that the V.A. should have known the patient was dangerous. Mrs. Lipari also filed suit against the V.A. claiming that the V.A. was negligent for failing to detain or commit the patient. The defendants moved to dismiss the complaints, but the Court denied the motion.

The Court held first, following *Tarasoff* and *McIntosh*, that there is a duty to protect that would apply in Nebraska. It further found, following paragraph 315, that the duty exists even where no specific victim has been threatened. Foreseeable violence, the Court said, is not limited to identified, specific victims, but may involve a class of persons at risk.

The Court also held that a psychotherapist "is not subject to liability for placing his patient in a less restrictive environment, so long as he uses due care in assessing the risks of such placement" (8, p. 193). The Court made clear its understanding that there were risks associated with placing patients in less restrictive settings, but it said that these risks were justified by the benefits deriving to patients, provided that the professionals involved had used reasonable care in making these decisions. The Court acknowledged that it is difficult to predict dangerousness, and that a bad outcome was not evidence of negligence.

The factual question of whether the V.A. was negligent in its treatment was never litigated. The federal government settled out of Court for over $200,000.

Comment: The published clinical data are rather sparse and unclear. The time relationship between first hospitalization, first day care, and buying the shotgun is not stated. The report does not state whether the treating clinicians knew that the patient owned a gun, or how dangerous they thought he was, or how thoroughly they evaluated his potential dangerousness.

This case, which extends liability to situations in which a specific victim is not named, involved a patient who was hospitalized and then treated in a day program. This case does not involve a patient in outpatient psychotherapy. The element of control over the patient, which paragraph 315 requires, is more clearly present for a patient in day treatment than for one who is only a psychotherapy patient.

In *Petersen v. Washington* (9), Supreme Court of the State of Washington, 1983, the plaintiff was injured when her car was struck by the car of a patient recently discharged from the state hospital. She charged negligence, claiming that the psychiatrist should have protected her from the dangerous propensities of the patient. Five days after being discharged, the patient ran a red light, apparently travelling between 50 and 60 miles per hour and under the influence of drugs. Four weeks earlier the patient had cut off one of his own testicles and been admitted to a state hospital. He gave a history of using angel dust just prior to his partial emasculation. He was treated at the hospital for three weeks with thiothixene, and he appeared to have a complete resolution of his psychosis. However, returning to the hospital from a pass on the day prior to his discharge, he was apprehended by hospital security personnel for reckless driving. Nevertheless, the psychiatrist did not petition for involuntary commitment, but discharged the patient.

At some later time, this patient raped a woman and murdered both her parents. At that time he was examined by two different psychiatrists who said he was schizophrenic, and this evidence was admitted in *Petersen* as bearing on the question of diagnosis. At trial, the treating psychiatrist testified that the patient was potentially dangerous, that he was liable to use angel dust again, and that he was unlikely to take his prescribed medicine.

The jury returned a verdict for the plaintiff.

On appeal, the Court chose to follow *Lipari*. It held that the doctor "incurred a duty to take reasonable precautions to protect anyone who might foreseeably be endangered by the patient's drug-related mental problems" (9, p. 237). The Court affirmed the verdict, finding that the State had a duty to protect this plaintiff, and that the psychiatrist had acted negligently in failing to take some action that would have better protected her.

In *Hedlund v. Orange County* (10), Supreme Court of California, 1983, a mother brought suit on her own behalf and on behalf of her son, charging that the defendant's psychotherapists had been negligent in failing to warn her that she was in danger from one of their patients. The victim was in couples therapy, along with the same man with whom she lived. When she was not present, he told the therapist that he planned to injure her. He subsequently used a shotgun to injure her. Her son was sitting next to her at the time and she threw herself across his body to protect him. The mother did not allege that her son was physically harmed; she sued for emotional damage.

The defendants argued that the son's claim for damages did not state a legally sufficient cause of action; but the Court disagreed. Without deciding what bystanders could be included, this Court, which had decided *Tarasoff* in 1976, held that the duty does extend to the young child of a threatened victim. When a patient makes a threat, injury to the victim's young child is also foreseeable because of the close relationship between mother and child.

Comment: The facts are presented sketchily, because of the legal posture of the case, so it is difficult to make much clinical sense out of this. The case report does not state what threats the patient made, or how thoroughly the therapists explored these threats. Nor does the report describe the patient's past history of violence, problems with impulse control, or drug or alcohol abuse.

This is another example of an identified victim for whom violence was held to be foreseeable. The precedent set by this decision is that the son, who was not threatened, was held to be a foreseeable victim, as well.

TARASOFF IS A DUTY, BUT NOT IN THIS CASE

No Identified Victim

In *Thompson v. County of Alameda* (11), 1980, the California Supreme Court held that the county was not negligent in releasing a juvenile delinquent who threatened to kill a child in the neighborhood, and who then killed a five-year-old boy within 24 hours of his release. The Court found that decisions to release are immune from liability. On the *Tarasoff* issue, the Court held that there is no affirmative duty to warn of the release of someone who has made "nonspecific threats of harm directed at nonspecific victims" (11, p. 735).

In *Leedy v. Hartnett* (12), 1981, a U.S. District Court in Pennsylvania held that the V.A. owed no duty to two people who were beaten by an alcoholic veteran recently discharged from a V.A. hospital. Although the veteran was staying in the home of the victims, the Court held that they were not foreseeable victims. The Court specifically declined to follow *Lipari*, and granted summary judgment for the hospital.

In *Holmes v. Wampler* (13), 1982, a victim who was stabbed by a discharged state hospital patient brought suit in a U.S. District court in Virginia for a civil rights violation. The patient had been released five weeks earlier. The stabbing was unprovoked. The plaintiff did not allege that the defendant psychiatrist knew or had any reason to know that the patient was dangerous to the victim. The suit was dismissed with prejudice, meaning this was the Court's final word.

In *Furr v. Spring Grove State Hospital* (14), 1982, Maryland Appeals Court, a patient who had a history of committing unnatural sexual acts on boys underwent a forensic evaluation and voluntarily committed himself to the hospital as part of a plea bargain in a criminal case. He subsequently escaped from the hospital, then returned to the hospital briefly, left again, and one week later committed brutal sex acts on an 11-year-old boy and murdered him. Following *Thompson,* the Court found that the doctors had no duty to warn because there was no foreseeable victim. Summary judgment was granted in favor of the defendants.

Control Not Sufficiently Present

In *Hasenei v. U.S.* (15), U.S. District Court, Maryland, 1982, Mr. and Mrs. Hasenei sued for damages when their car collided head-on with a car driven by a veteran who was a patient at a V.A. outpatient psychiatric clinic. The patient, who died in the accident, was driving on the wrong side of the road with his lights off, and had a blood alcohol level of 250 mg per liter—well above the legal standard for intoxication.

The dead man had a five year history of alcoholism and a history of alcohol-related violence, including threatening his wife with a knife, fighting in the hope of being killed, burning a barroom, and smashing a liquor store window. In January 1976, he was hospitalized with diagnoses of schizophrenia and alcoholism. He was treated with chlorpromazine, 1600 mg per day, which apparently helped control his drinking, and he attended Alcoholics Anonymous. He was discharged in April, and given an outpatient appointment that he did not keep.

On August 9, 1976, 12 days prior to the accident, he did come to the clinic stating that he had been dry until late June. At that time his four-year-old son had been killed by a car while in the patient's charge. Thereafter, the patient blamed himself, became depressed, and began to drink. However, at the clinic he appeared to be in good contact, neither psychotic nor intoxicated. His wife, who accompanied him, told a social worker that her husband was not drinking heavily, and that he was not homicidal or suicidal. The patient was started on thioridazine and given a one month follow-up appointment.

At trial, plaintiffs claimed that the psychiatrist was grossly negligent: in not trying to persuade the patient to go into the hospital voluntarily; in not hospitalizing him involuntarily; in changing his chlorpromazine to thioridazine; in not giving him an appointment before one month; and in not reporting the patient to the Department of Motor Vehicles as a dangerous driver so that his license would be suspended.

The V.A. defended on the grounds that the psychiatrist was not negligent; that the patient was not committable; that the accident was not proximately caused by the medical treatment; and that reporting the patient to the Department of Motor Vehicles was illegal under Pennsylvania law and breached the patient's confidentiality.

In considering its judgment, the Court made extensive reference to paragraph 315, pointing out that none of the previous *Tarasoff* cases had defined what it is about the patient-therapist relationship that brings it within the 315 rule. The Court found that the existence of this special duty must rest on the actor's right or ability to control the other. Clearly, the opinion goes on, under ordinary circumstances, the outpatient psychotherapeutic relationship is not such a relationship.

The Court found that the psychiatrist had raised the question of hospitalization, but the patient had been adamantly against it. Even the plaintiffs agreed that the patient did not meet standards for civil commitment. The Court noted that the patient had not taken his chlorpromazine since leaving the hospital, so that even if the psychiatrist had not changed the patient's medicine, there was no reason to believe that the patient would have taken it. Concerning his driving, the Court said that suspending his license would have been ineffective, since a man who will drive drunk on the wrong side of the road with his lights off is unlikely to be deterred from driving by loss of his license. The Court saw no basis for predicting the patient's dangerousness with any reasonable degree of medical certainty.

Based on these facts, the Court found the psychiatrist did not have a duty to these plaintiffs. The Court further found that the psychiatrist had not been negligent, and it entered judgment for the defendant.

In *Brady v. Hopper* (16), U.S. District Court, Colorado, 1983, the plaintiffs were all men who had been shot by one of the defendant's patients, John Hinckley. Hinckley's parents brought their son to the psychiatrist because they were concerned about his behavior, including a purported recent suicide attempt by drug overdose. The psychiatrist treated his patient with diazepam and biofeedback, and told the parents that the patient should be on his own. The plaintiffs alleged that this treatment made the patient worse, and potentially more dangerous.

The patient subsequently left Colorado, and traveled to Washington, D.C., where he attempted to assassinate President Reagan, and did shoot and injure the plaintiffs. Prior to this action the patient had no history of violence except to himself. He had never been arrested, had never been hospitalized because of violence toward others, and he had not appeared to be a danger to others. He had, however, been preoccupied with the movie *Taxi Driver*, and he appeared to identify with the protagonist-killer.

The plaintiff's complaint alleged that the psychiatrist's treatment aggravated Hinckley's condition; that the psychiatrist should have sought consultation; and that he should have warned Hinckley's parents and law enforcement personnel about John Hinckley's dangerousness. The defendant moved to dismiss the complaint, arguing that he had no way of knowing that Hinckley would be dangerous, and in the absence of threats to a specific identifiable person he had no duty to warn or take other action to control the patient's behavior. He argued further that the patient did not meet standards for involuntary hospitalization, and that Colorado law prevented him from breaching the patient's confidentiality.

Plaintiffs argued that there is a duty to control a patient's behavior if the psychiatrist could reasonably be expected to know that the patient was dangerous to others, whether these others were named or not. They argued further that the psychiatrist did control the patient, citing as evidence the fact that the gave the patient diazepam and biofeedback. Furthermore, they argued that the psychiatrist had a duty to control the patient's potential violence because it was foreseeable, based on the patient's preoccupation with the movie *Taxi Driver*.

In ruling on the motion, the Court focused not on whether the therapist-patient relationship gave rise to a broad duty to protect the public, but rather on whether the pyschiatrist was obligated to protect these particular plaintiffs from this particular harm. It said that the answer to this question depended upon whether the harm to the plaintiffs was foreseeable.

For purposes of deciding the issue, the Court assumed the psychiatrist's treatment of Hinckley fell below the applicable standards of care. Nevertheless, the Court concluded that the plaintiffs' injuries were not foreseeable. Consequently, the psychiatrist bore no responsibility for them. The Court further concluded that there was no relationship between the defendant and the victims from which a duty might follow. Finally, the Court said there were cogent reasons to limit the scope of the therapist's liability. "To impose upon those in the counseling professions an ill-defined "duty to control" would require therapists to be ultimately responsible for the actions of their patients... Human behavior is simply too unpredictable, and the field of psychotherapy presently too inexact, to so greatly expand the scope of therapists' liability" (16, p. 1339). Declining to find the psychiatrist legally responsible, the Court dismissed the complaint.

Comment: The Court did not imply that the psychiatrist had been negligent. Its statement that it assumed negligence was required because this was a motion to dismiss. On a motion to dismiss, the Court must assume a view of the facts most favorable to the plaintiff, and then consider the question of law. Such a view, in this case, would assume the psychiatrist was negligent.

REFUSALS TO FOLLOW *TARASOFF*

In *Shaw v. Glickman* (17), Maryland Court of Appeals, 1980, Dr. Shaw was at home in his own bed at 2 A.M. with a woman who was separated from her husband. The husband broke into Dr. Shaw's home, and as the Court described the scene, "Both were nude. [The husband] obviously believing he had been cuckolded, discharged five bullets into the body of Dr. Shaw. Either [the husband] was a poor shot or an excellent one, because none of the wounds were fatal" (17, p. 627).

Dr. Shaw and the dissolving couple had all been patients of the same psychiatric team. Dr. Shaw sued the team for negligently failing to warn him that one of their patients, that is, the husband, was violent and unstable and presented a danger to him. In a therapy session, the wife told her husband that she had been involved with someone else. According to the wife, the therapist later told her husband the identity of this person, who was in fact the plaintiff, Dr. Shaw. The husband was known to have a gun but there was no allegation that he had ever specifically threatened Dr. Shaw.

The trial Court granted summary judgment for the psychiatric team on the grounds that Dr. Shaw assumed the risk of injury because he voluntarily placed himself in a potentially dangerous situation. Dr. Shaw appealed this decision to the Appeals Court, which found that *Tarasoff* did not apply in this case, since the husband had not threatened or expressed any animosity toward the plaintiff. The fact that the husband carried a gun did not imply danger to Dr. Shaw. The Court also noted that the therapists had a duty grounded in the Hippocratic Oath and in statutory law to preserve confidentiality.

Comment: Subsequently, Dr. Shaw married the woman in this case. The husband, who had been convicted of assault, paid Dr. Shaw $20,000 in settlement of Dr. Shaw's claim against the husband for injuries resulting from the shooting.

In *Doyle v. U.S.* (18), U.S. District Court in California, 1982, a veteran was discharged from service one month after being discharged from a psychiatric hospital. After leaving the service he traveled 1,000 miles, killing a man two days later. The court said there was no foreseeable victim, and that the killing occurred too far away and too long after his discharge for the medical treatment to have been the proximate cause. The case was dismissed.

In *Peck v. Counseling Service of Addison County* (19), County Court of Vermont, 1983, the patient was a 31-year-old epileptic man who had been treated by neurologists and psychiatrists for years, and who had exhibited impulsive, dangerous antisocial behavior. After three years of treatment with the defendant counseling center and the counselor, the patient left the area and went to live in a halfway house. He was asked to leave the halfway house after a fight with another resident, and he moved back in with his parents with whom he did not get along. He again began counseling with the counselor whom he had not seen for two years.

His father suggested that the patient lie to Social Security in order to get benefits to which he was not entitled. When the son became angry and refused, the father told him he was sick and belonged in a hospital. The patient then took his belongings and left, and went to the counselor. She helped him find a place to live. The next day he told her about the argument, and that he was angry at this father. Five days later he told her he would probably burn down his father's barn. They discussed the matter further and the patient assured the counselor that he would not carry out this threat. She believed him. The next day he burned the barn down.

The counselor had a Masters in Education degree, and was responsible for consulting her supervising psychiatrist as needed.

In this case, she wrote a note about the threat, but did not alert the psychiatrist. She had spoken to the patient's former counselors, but not to his most recent physician. She had written for his past medical records, but they had not yet come. Therefore, she did not know that he was under "heavy medication and that patient control was difficult, both in controlling his epileptic seizure problems and his emotional problems." There was no evidence that she checked to see whether he was complying with his treatment regimen.

The plaintiffs, who were the patient's parents and the owners of the burned barn, sued the counseling center for the damage to their barn. They claimed that the defendant should have known that their son was dangerous to them and their property, that they failed to notify them or others who could have taken steps to protect them, that they failed to further evaluate the patient's dangerousness, and that as a result of this negligence, the client burned down the plaintiff's barn, which was worth $137,526.13.

The Court found, as a matter of fact, that a reasonably prudent counseling service would have a system for cross-referencing between physician and non-physician for patients with severe medical problems; that the counselor should have consulted with a supervising counselor, with the psychiatrist, or with the past treating physician; or that the counselor should have taken a more complete history concerning the threat, including how often he had the idea, when he first had it, how long he had it, and how he would go about implementing it.

The Court further found that the counseling service was negligent in not having the recent medical history, and in not having a cross-reference system. It said that the counselor acted in good faith, but her belief was based on inadequate information and inadequate consultation. In finding that the defendants should have recognized the substantial risk that the son was capable of carrying out his threat, the Court cited the following factors: anger at the father over a six day period; recent history of impulsive violence; specific threat; history of noncompliance with treatment; recent history of epileptic seizures; and history of alcohol abuse. Finally, the Court found that the father's own negligent conduct toward his son contributed to 50 percent of the damages.

As a matter of law, the Court held that if *Tarasoff* were the law in Vermont, the counseling service would have had a duty to warn the Pecks. However, the Court declined to be the agent by which a *Tarasoff* duty was introduced into Vermont law. The Court dismissed the complaint, and it explicitly left to the legislature or the Appeals Court the task of deciding whether Vermont law should include a duty to protect. The case is currently on appeal to the Supreme Court of Vermont.

Comment: In spite of the fact that the judge thought the standard of care was negligent, he declined to find the defendants negligent, because there was no basis in Vermont law for them to recover on their complaint.

In *Hopewell v. Adibempe* (20), Court of Common Pleas, Allegheny County, Pennsylvania, 1981, the plaintiff was a patient of the defendant psychiatrist who worked in a community mental health center. The patient told her psychiatrist that she would "blow up and hurt somebody very seriously if the harassment" on the job did not stop. Without having prior written consent from the patient, the psychiatrist sent the following letter to the woman's personnel director:

"In the course of a psychiatric interview which took place in my office, ... the above-named reported feelings of being so enraged about her work situation that she 'will blow up and hurt somebody very seriously if the harassment does not stop.'

"This information is being relayed to you because there is a legal precedent requiring it and is not to be taken as an estimate of the probability that the threat will actually be carried out. It is, however, important that the person or persons at risk be notified. In this case I believe that her immediate supervisor should know of this letter."

The letter further contained the following stamped endorsement, "THIS INFORMATION HAS BEEN DISCLOSED TO YOU FROM RECORDS WHOSE CONFIDENTIALITY IS PROTECTED BY STATE LAW. STATE REGULATIONS PROHIBIT YOU FROM MAKING ANY FURTHER DISCLOSURES OF

THIS INFORMATION WITHOUT THE PRIOR CONSENT OF THE PERSON IN RESPECT TO WHOM IT PERTAINS."

The Court noted that *Tarasoff* raised the question of a duty, but said that in the state where the plaintiff and defendant lived, the law effectively eliminated the *Tarasoff* duty by striking the balance in favor of confidentiality through the passage of an appropriate statute. The Court said that the psychiatrist had clearly violated this law. Accordingly, the Court found the defendant liable for having breached the defendant's confidentality, but the Court declined to express an opinion on the amount of damages that should be imposed.

Comment: The defendant was held liable, not for breach of a *Tarasoff* duty that the Court said did not exist in that jurisdiction, but for breach of confidentiality. However, there are important clinical facts missing from the published account. We do not know if the psychiatrist discussed his proposed course of action with the patient and failed to gain her consent, or whether he wrote the letter without discussing it. As will be reported in Chapter Four, it is common for psychiatrists who warn to also report that they have compromised their clinical judgment at some time in their professional lives. From the tone of the letter, it appears that the psychiatrist was motivated primarily by a concern to fulfill a legal obligation, rather than by his clinical assessment of what was called for, and that he may well have felt that his clinical judgment was compromised. In such a case the psychiatrist is likely not to discuss the proposed course of action, but to simply go forward. Whether these speculations are correct or not, this case supports Roth's conviction of the importance of gaining informed consent from the patient before acting (21).

CONCLUSION

It is difficult to discern a single legal doctrine emerging from the cases decided to date. One conclusion does seem justified: most Courts have held that, absent a foreseeable victim, there is no duty to protect. It is noteworthy that there have been so few published cases in the 10 years since *Tarasoff*. Therapists' initial fears that

Tarasoff would lead to a spate of litigation have not, apparently, been borne out.

Psychiatrists were originally most concerned that the *Tarasoff* duty would interfere with the relationship between the psycho-therapist and the patient, a relationship which typically involves the psychiatrist and an outpatient. If we examine the outpatient cases as a group, a striking finding emerges: No Court outside California has applied the *Tarasoff* doctrine to a case involving outpatient psychotherapy, and then gone on to find liability on the facts. In *McIntosh* (3) the Court said there was a duty, but found the psychiatrist not negligent. *Lipari* (8) involved a patient in day care. In *Shaw* (17), *Hasenei* (15), and *Brady* (16), the Court said *Tarasoff* did not apply because there was no threat to the victim. In *Peck* (19), the Court said that *Tarasoff* was not the law in its jurisdiction. *Hedlund* (10) and *Jablonski* (6) are California cases.

There have been eight cases involving discharged inpatients in which the *Tarasoff* duty has been raised as a cause of action. Seven have been decided. In five of these seven cases, *Thompson* (11), *Leedy* (12), *Holmes* (13), *Furr* (14), and *Doyle* (18), the Courts found that the victim was not foreseeable and that the defendant therefore had no duty to protect. In all of these cases there was no question as to the standard of the defendant's care. In *Petersen* (9), the defendant was found to be negligent, but the Court suggested not that he might have taken some unusual action to protect the public, but rather that he might have petitioned for commitment of his patient—a suggestion with which, on the facts, many psychiatrists would agree. *Davis* (4), is the only case in which a psychiatrist was found negligent for failing to protect a victim, although there was no question of substandard care. In 10 years, this is the only published case in the United States in which a psychiatrist was found negligent for failing to warn in the absence of any allegation of substandard care.

Commentators, for example, Appelbaum (22), have been con-cerned about the expansion of liability for failure to protect, citing the *Lipari* (8) decision as one example. Only one Court has followed *Lipari*, and several have explicitly rejected this expansion of the duty (4, 11). The one case that followed *Lipari* found the psychiatrist negligent in not committing the patient, so that as a practical matter there was no expansion; the psychiatrist was faulted for failing to do what psychiatrists have always done with patients who are potentially violent and mentally ill: committed them.

In summary, this chapter illustrates that there have been only four published cases outside California in which the Courts have ruled that there is a *Tarasoff* duty to which a defendant should be held. The four cases are *McIntosh* (3) in New Jersey, *Lipari* (8) in Nebraska, *Davis* (4) in Michigan, and *Petersen* (9) in the state of Washington. Although there have been no published *Tarasoff* cases in 46 states and the District of Columbia, most commentators agree that all psychotherapists should practice as if the *Tarasoff* duty to protect is the law. The duty to protect is, in effect, at present a national standard of practice, in spite of the fact that it is not the law in most jurisdictions, and in spite of the fact that the duty itself is subject to different interpretations by different Courts.

The consensus that there exists a duty to protect that devolves upon all therapists has led to a developing communality of concern among all therapists, not merely those in jurisdictions in which *Tarasoff* is the law. The impact of the *Tarasoff* duty is a subject on which there has been wide debate, but relatively little information. The major source of the information we do have, a survey by Givelber and his colleagues, is presented in the next chapter.

References

1. *Restatement (Second) of Torts:* #315

2. Prosser WL, Wade JW, Schwartz V: Torts: *Cases and Materials*, 7th Ed., Foundation Press, Mineola, NY, 1982

3. *McIntosh v. Milano*, 403 A.2d 500 (N.J. Supr. Ct. 1979)

4. *Davis v. Lhim*, Mich. Wayne County Circuit Court, No. 77-726989 NM (June 11, 1981)

5. *Chrite v. U.S.*, 564F Supp. 341, (1983)

6. *Jablonski v. U.S.*, 712 F.2d 391 (9th Cir. 1983)

7. *MacDonald v. Clinger*, App. Div., 446N.Y.S.2d 801 (1982)

8. *Lipari v. Sears, Roebuck & Co.*, 497 F. Supp. 185 (D. Neb. 1980)

9. *Petersen v. Washington*, 671 P.2d 23 0 (Wash. 1983)

10. *Hedlund v. Orange County*, 669 P.2d 41 (Cal. 1983)

11. *Thompson v. County of Alameda*, 167 Cal. Rptr. 70 (1980)

12. *Leedy v. Hartnett*, 519 F. Supp. 1125 (1981)

13. *Holmes v. Wampler*, 546 F. Supp. 500 (EO VA 11 1982)

14. *Furr v. Spring Grove State Hospital*, 53 Md. App.474, 454 A2d 414 (1983)

15. *Hasenei v. U.S.*, 541 F. Supp. 999 (D. Md. 1982)

16. *Brady v. Hopper*, 570 F. Supp. 1333 (D. Colo. 1983)

17. *Shaw v. Glickman*, Md. App., 415A.2d 625, (1980)

18. *Doyle v. U.S.*, 530 F. Supp. 1278 (C.D. Cal. 1982)

19. *Peck v. Counseling Service of Addison County, Inc.*, Vt. Addison Sup Ct, No. S114-80Ac (January 17, 1983)

20. *Hopewell v. Adibempe*, No. GD78-82756, Civil Division, Court of Common Pleas of Allegheny County, Pennsylvania, June 1, 1981

21. Roth LH, Meisel A: Dangerousness, confidentiality, and the duty to warn. Am J Psychiatry 134:508–511, 1977

22. Appelbaum PS: The expansion of liability for patients' violent acts. Hosp Community Psychiatry 35:13, 1984

3

The *Tarasoff* Controversy: A Summary of Findings From an Empirical Study of Legal, Ethical, and Clinical Issues

Daniel J.Givelber, J.D.
William J. Bowers, Ph.D.
Carolyn L. Blitch, M.A.

3

The *Tarasoff* Controversy: A Summary of Findings From an Empirical Study of Legal, Ethical, and Clinical Issues

In its *Tarasoff* decision, the California Supreme Court ruled that a psychotherapist has a legal duty to exercise reasonable care to protect potential victims from violent patients (1). The therapist must respond when he or she concludes, or in the exercise of reasonable professional care, should conclude, that a patient poses a threat of imminent violence toward another. If the therapist fails to meet his or her obligation and the patient harms a foreseeable victim, then the therapist may be liable in money damages to the victim.

Tarasoff extended a traditional principle of law to a new situation. With few exceptions, the law requires all of us to behave reasonably to avoid injuring others by our actions. Some of us (for example, parents, bus companies, innkeepers) have the additional obligation to act affirmatively to prevent others from harming those within our care (for example, children, passengers, guests). In a very few situations the opposite is also true: we must control those within our care (for instance, our children) to prevent them from injuring others (for instance, an unsuspecting babysitter). If we fail to meet these obligations and, as a result,

This work was supported by the National Institute of Mental Health, Grant Number RO 1 MH 32439-011.

someone is injured, then we are required to compensate the injured person. This body of law—known as tort law—is enforced typically by private parties suing one another in Court. The injured party brings a lawsuit and, if he or she prevails, can secure a judgment from the Court requiring that the injurer pay for the harm caused.

In the *Tarasoff* case, the legal process was truncated by an out-of-Court settlement between the parties. The effect of the *Tarasoff* decision was to reinstate the Tarasoff family's legal complaint, which the defendants had sought to dismiss, and give them an opportunity to prove their allegations at trial. The trial never occurred; the parties settled out of Court. What has not been settled is the debate surrounding the wisdom of the *Tarasoff* rule and its effect on therapeutic practice.

The *Tarasoff* decision has been attacked on a number of grounds, including the following: a) the decision rested on the false view that there were valid professional standards that enabled therapists to predict future violence; b) in effect, the decision imposed a requirement to warn potential victims; the very existence of this requirement, and compliance with it, would compromise the confidentiality necessary to successful psychotherapy; and c) the decision raised a therapist's obligation to the public over his or her obligation to the patient, thereby compromising central professional ethical precepts. As a result of these conflicts, the *Tarasoff* decision might discourage therapists from treating potentially violent patients; or lead therapists to overreact to nonserious threats; or lead therapists to respond incorrectly to serious threats; or drive patients away from therapy. This could, in turn, lead to increased violence and reduced public safety (2). Thus, *Tarasoff* extended judicial intrusion from public institutions to private psychotherapeutic practice, and threatened therapists with tort suits based upon their exercise of an ability that they insisted they did not possess.

While some of the controversy surrounding the decision reflects a conflict in values and ideology, some of the contentions can be resolved empirically. We undertake this task in this chapter.

There has been one previous survey of the impact of the *Tarasoff* rule on practitioners (3). In 1977, Wise surveyed psychiatrists and psychologists in California, and achieved a 34 percent response rate. Her average respondent was a 45-year-old male in private practice with a psychoanalytic outlook, treating 240 different patients each year. Over 80 percent had seen a patient thought to be dangerous, and the average number of potentially dangerous patients seen each year was reported to be 14. Virtually all the respondents knew about *Tarasoff*.

Most therapists said that their patients generally believed that confidentiality was absolute, but they themselves believed that confidentiality should be broken under some circumstances. However, few therapists reported that they discussed confidentiality with patients.

After *Tarasoff* there was a substantial increase in the number of potential victims warned. Therapists reported more discussion of confidentiality and dangerousness with both patients and colleagues. Many therapists reported that they had lowered the threshold at which they became concerned about violence, and the threshold at which they explored potential violence with patients. Once patients knew that breach of confidentiality was a possibility, 25 percent were noted to be reluctant to discuss violent tendencies, and 25 percent of therapists said that at least one patient had terminated because of this concern.

A majority of therapists reported that they were increasingly anxious and fearful of lawsuits. Sixteen percent reported that, since *Tarasoff*, they have avoided probing dangerousness. Wise concluded that attitudes of therapists had changed, with most being more responsible about dealing with possible violence, while a minority tried to avoid the issue. The results of the study are broadly consistent with the results of ours.

Our findings are presented in five sections, each of which deals with a particular aspect of the *Tarasoff* case. In the first section, we are concerned with knowledge and beliefs about *Tarasoff*: which therapists know about *Tarasoff*, when they believe it applies, and what they believe it requires of them. In the second section, we deal with the issue of predicting potential violence: what factors therapists use in determining that a patient may be dangerous to others, and the degree to which uniform standards for such predictions exist. In the third section, we examine the interventions employed with potentially dangerous patients. The fourth section concerns the reported consequences of therapists warning potential victims of their patients. The fifth section addresses the issue of the impact of beliefs, both legal and ethical, on psychotherapists' attitudes and clinical practices.

The data for this study comes from a questionnaire sent to a sample of psychiatrists, psychologists, and social workers in the eight largest metropolitan areas of the United States. The instrument was specifically designed to measure the effects of the *Tarasoff* decision upon the practice of psychotherapy (4).

Of the 2,875 therapists sent questionnaires, 59.5 percent (1,722) responded. Returns were fairly equally distributed over the eight metropolitan areas, indicating no substantial differences in response by location.

Although the California Supreme Court spoke in terms of therapists generally, we treat it as a matter of sociological faith that professional differences matter, and therefore present the results for each profession separately. Where appropriate, we also discuss differences that are related to the settings in which patients are seen. We distinguish between Californians and others to illustrate one of our major findings—that tort rulings, directed to and enforced by private parties, may influence behavior even where they are not "the law." The text is organized by statements of our findings. With respect to each statement, we address the reasons that the issue is important, and present our analysis and conclusions regarding the data.

KNOWLEDGE AND BELIEFS ABOUT *TARASOFF*

1. *Tarasoff* is well known among therapists, particularly Californians and psychiatrists.

Virtually every psychiatrist (96 percent), and 90 percent of psychologists and social workers in California had heard of the decision by name, or had heard of a case "like it," but did not recognize the name (5). Yet psychiatrists from places other than California are not far behind—87 percent know the case by name, and another seven percent have heard of a case like it. The strong showing by psychiatrists should not obscure two other facts: 90 percent of California psychologists and social workers also know about the case, while almost 75 percent of out-of-state psychologists know about it, as do more than 50 percent of the non-California social workers. This data demonstrates that the Court and its critics were justified in believing that they were dealing with a decision that would be well known and, therefore, might have a substantial influence on therapeutic practice.

2. Most respondents understand correctly that *Tarasoff* applies when either a) therapists assess a patient as potentially violent, or b) as reasonable therapists, they should have assessed the patient in this manner.

We asked our respondents to indicate under what conditions *Tarasoff* imposes the duty to protect another: whenever the patient makes a threat; whenever a reasonable therapist would assess the patient as dangerous toward another; or whenever the therapist actually makes such an assessment. Ninety percent thought that the *Tarasoff* obligation applies *both* when a therapist actually believes someone is dangerous, and also when a reasonable therapist would believe this. They understood correctly the Court's statement in this regard.

3. Most therapists believe incorrectly that *Tarasoff* requires them to warn potential victims rather than to exercise reasonable care.

Among our respondents, more than 75 percent believe *Tarasoff* requires warning a victim, while only slightly more than 35 percent believe that it mandates the exercise of reasonable care. Furthermore, of those who believe *Tarasoff* requires warning a victim, approximately two-thirds believe that reasonable care is *not* required. Californians are 20 percent more likely than therapists from other states to believe that warning alone satisfies the

Tarasoff requirement. Psychiatrists outside of California are about 10 percent more likely than corresponding psychologists and social workers to make the same claim. Clearly, the majority of our therapists believe that warning a victim is the appropriate response to a *Tarasoff* situation, with Californians and psychiatrists from other states most likely to "misstate" the formal holding of *Tarasoff.*

ASSESSMENT OF IMMINENT VIOLENCE

4. Most therapists believe that they can make meaningful assessments of potential future violence of their patients.

Our respondents proved to be rather more confident about their ability to identify future violence than the arguments of the *Tarasoff* critics suggested. When asked to indicate the strongest prediction they would be willing to make with respect to the possibility that a non-institutionalized patient of theirs might physically harm another, only five percent of our respondents felt that there was "no way to predict" such behavior, and over three-quarters felt that they could make a prediction ranging from "probable" to "certain."

5. Over 85 percent of our therapists cite threats of violence, a history of violence, or current or recent acts of violence as influential in their assessment of a patient as potentially violent.

We asked therapists to "list or otherwise indicate . . . what factors were influential in your determination that the patient or client was likely to physically attack or harm others" in the "most recent case in which you believed a patient was likely to physically attack or harm someone else." We coded the open-ended responses to this question into 19 general factor categories, the relative frequencies of which are shown in Table 1.

The results of this analysis show that our respondents attach a great deal of importance to behavior involving or threatening violence in assessing potential dangerousness to others. At least

Table 1. Assessing Potential Dangerousness to Others

Type of Factor	Percent of Cases in Which Cited	Number of Cases in Which Cited
Violent or Assaultive Factor		
History of violent or assaultive behavior	39	471
Threats of future violent assaultive behavior	36	437
Current or recent violent or assaultive behavior	19	227
Behavior		
Hostile or aggressive behavior	15	181
History of hostile or aggressive behavior	4	44
Behavior neither violent nor hostile or aggressive	17	211
History of behavior, neither violent nor hostile or aggressive	2	25
Emotional or Cognitive States		
Violent fantasies, ideation, or feelings	10	119
Hostile feelings or angry ideation	11	140
Other cognitive or emotional states	27	331
Social or Environmental Stressors		
Hostile, disturbed, or inadequate relations with others	13	155
History of hostile, disturbed, or inadequate relations with others	5	64
Environmental or situational stressors	12	147
Clinical Diagnosis, Evaluation, or Judgment		
Psychotic diagnosis or label	22	272
History of psychotic diagnosis or label	1	11
Nonpsychotic diagnosis or label	25	311
History of nonpsychotic diagnosis or label	2	28
Resistant or nonresponsive to treatment	6	67
Clinical evidence or general evaluation	11	139

one reference to a history of violent assaultive behavior is reported in 39 percent of all cases. Threats of future violence are the second most frequently cited indicators, with 36 percent of all respondents listing at least one threat. Current or recent violence is represented in 19 percent of all cases. Other factors that are not violence-related are mentioned considerably less frequently.

Our questionnaire also asked respondents whether there had been an explicit verbal threat in the most recent case. Including data from this item, 85 percent of our respondents mention at least one violence-related factor in their assessment. Verbal threats are mentioned in more than one-half of the cases. In 27 percent of all cases, they are mentioned in conjunction with either current or past violent behavior. In 29 percent of all cases, they are mentioned without any other violence-related factor.

6. Most respondents rely on the same factors for assessment purposes regardless of their profession, the setting in which the patient is seen, or the location of their practice.

There are few differences in assessment criteria cited by different professionals. Psychiatrists are about 10 percent more likely to report verbal threats than are others, but they do not differ in the extent to which they cite current or recent violent behavior or combinations of these factors. Assessment criteria also do not differ substantially by the setting in which the patient is seen, although, as might be expected, a history of violence is reported somewhat more frequently for inpatients than for those in outpatient treatment. Jurisdictional differences are negligible.

Our data further suggest that therapists use similar standards to evaluate cases in which these factors appear. For instance, cases containing verbal threats were about twice as likely as other cases to be considered highly serious and highly likely to result in injury. There were no substantial differences in these rates for different professions, settings, or locations.

The lack of significant differences among these subgroups suggests a national and cross-professional consistency in the assessment of potential for future violence. They tend to support the

California Supreme Court's approach in two respects. First, it may be appropriate to treat therapists as a group in terms of dangerousness assessment, rather than to deal with each professional group separately. Second, the consistency in patterns of assessment factors suggests that therapists everywhere may approach the issue of assessment in similar ways.

7. Most therapists believe that colleagues would agree with their assessment that a given patient is potentially violent.

One final piece of evidence also suggests that in addition to using similar assessment standards, therapists also perceive these standards to be widely shared by their professional colleagues. Seven out of 10 respondents believed that 90 to 100 percent of their colleagues would agree with their conclusion that the patient was potentially violent. The responses were remarkably consistent across profession and by location with the exception of California psychiatrists, who displayed less confidence in the agreement of their colleagues than did those practicing elsewhere. Since this is the very group most sensitized to *Tarasoff*, the finding hints at the possibility that exposure to the case, or perhaps the criticism of it, may affect attitudes and beliefs respecting evaluation of potential violence. However, even one-fourth of this group believed that everyone would agree with their evaluation of the patient, and another three-eighths (37 percent) believed that 90 percent of their colleagues would agree. Thus, therapists, at least, appear to believe that there are professional standards for evaluating dangerousness or, at a minimum, that dangerousness is a little like hard core obscenity in that they "know it when they see it," even if they can't define it.

ACTIONS EMPLOYED WITH POTENTIALLY VIOLENT PATIENTS

8. Warning a victim is not common. It occurs in only 15 percent of all cases. Discussing the matter in treatment and documenting potentially violent behavior are the most frequent responses to the potentially violent patient.

We asked therapists to indicate the actions they had taken or recommended taking with regard to the patient they had assessed as potentially violent in the "most recent case." Here we presented the therapist with a list of 16 actions and an opportunity to write in any additional ones he or she might also have recommended or employed.

For the analysis of the data, we grouped all of the actions reported into seven major categories: treatment; documentation; consultation; notification of non-therapists; hospitalization; declining, transferring, or terminating treatment; and actions related to changing the status or environment of the patient. The major headings and the individual actions included under each are presented in Table 2.

Of these seven types of actions, treatment and documentation are the two most frequently recommended or employed by our respondents; 76 percent of all therapists take up the problem of potential violence in therapy, and 55 percent make notes in the patient's record concerning potential violence. The least frequently mentioned interventions are decline, terminate, or transfer treatment (six percent), and change status or environment (one percent). Consultations occur in about 30 percent of all cases. Voluntary hospitalization and notifying family or friends are more common (26 percent and 33 percent, respectively) than involuntary hospitalization and notification of other non-therapists (20 percent and 12 percent, respectively). The intervention that our respondents are most likely to identify with *Tarasoff*, warning potential victims, is recommended or employed in only 15 percent of all cases.

There are few differences in the actions employed by different professionals. Psychiatrists are somewhat less likely to recommend treatment or seek independent consultations, and are somewhat more likely to recommend or employ involuntary hospitalization, alter medications, and include notes in the record. Social workers are more likely to decline or terminate treatment and to consult others. All other actions, including warning potential victims, are employed at about the same rate by psychiatrists, psychologists, and social workers.

Table 2. For Each Pattern of Assessment Factor Cited, Percent of Respondents who Recommended or Initiated Each Action

Recommended or Initiated Action	PERCENTAGE FOR EACH ACTION ASSESSMENT FACTOR			
	No Violent Behavior	Current History Violent Only	Threat Only	Current History and Threat
Treatment				
Took up in	74	77	75	79
More treatment	51	52	44	50
Practical advice	39	39	39	39
Alter medication	26	30	30	33
Change treatment plan	4	7	3	3
Document				
Note in record*	44	47	58	66
Document consultation	34	38	39	43
Consultation				
Independent evaluation	15	12	15	15
Psychological test	11	12	11	15
Consult others	8	10	9	8
Notify Non-Therapists				
Family or friends*	29	26	37	38
Potential victim*	9	6	21	19
Police*	2	5	10	11
Other public authorities*	10	11	9	16
Hospitalize				
Voluntary	25	21	29	27
Involuntary*	12	14	21	28
Decline, Terminate, or Transfer				
Decline or terminate treatment	5	6	7	6
Transfer to another therapist	2	3	3	2
Change Status or Environment				
Transfer to locked facility	1	—	—	—
Transfer from voluntary to involuntary status	—	—	1	1
Seclusion or observation	—	—	1	—
Change life situation	2	1	3	2
	N = 200	251	393	368

*$X^2 p < .05$

9. Warning a victim is virtually always accompanied by some other action on the part of the therapist.

Treatment and documentation of potentially violent behavior occur in 80 percent of all warning cases; treatment, documentation, and hospitalization occur in 43 percent of all such cases. Moreover, in 73 percent of these warning cases, the therapist also attempted to notify someone else—either friend or family, the police, or other public agencies. In fully 97 percent of the cases reported, warning a victim was accompanied by an attempt to notify at least one other non-therapist, or by an attempt at hospitalization.

Our data also indicate no major differences among the combinations of other actions recommended or taken by therapists in different professions or locations. It therefore appears that warning a victim is one of many responses to dangerous patients that may be added to a therapist's repertoire, but it does not appear to be used as a substitute for other actions.

10. Therapists treating patients in private practice are more likely to warn potential victims, and are less likely to initiate involuntary hospitalization or document for the record, than are those seeing patients in institutional settings.

Actions taken vary somewhat more by the setting in which a patient is seen. Treatment and voluntary hospitalization are more common responses to private outpatients than to inpatients or those seen in an institutional outpatient setting. Documenting potentially violent behavior, involuntary hospitalization, and notifying police and other public authorities are more frequently employed with patients seen in institutional settings. Warning potential victims is somewhat more likely to be employed with private outpatients than others, but differences are small. Warnings are issued in 13 percent of cases involving inpatients, 15 percent involving institutional outpatients, and 19 percent of private practice outpatients.

11. Therapists are more likely to notify third parties, involuntarily hospitalize patients, and document their actions, when the patient has made threats.

Table 2 shows the ways in which the kinds of factors cited in assessing potential violence are related to the types of interventions our respondents employ. Verbal threats are disproportionately associated with note taking, notifying family or friends or potential victims and police, and involuntary hospitalization. Furthermore, the percentages are approximately the same in cases where past or current violent behavior is also present, as in cases where verbal threats alone are cited. Thus, it appears to be the verbal threat and not some other combination of threats and violence-related behavior that accounts for these differences.

12. Therapists are most likely to warn potential victims when the patient has made an explicit verbal threat identifying the victim.

When we turn to the issue of which kinds of threats are associated with documentation, notifying non-therapists, and involuntary hospitalization, we find that verbal threats with specified victims are associated with a higher level of notifying family or friends and warning potential victims than are other verbal threats. This is, of course, hardly surprising, as it is difficult to warn victims who are not known to the therapist. The higher level of notifying among family or friends may also be partially explained by the likelihood that the victim is included among family and friends.

On the other hand, the rate of recommended involuntary hospitalization is slightly higher for verbal threats that do not name the victim than for those in which victims are specified. Similarly, there are no substantial differences in the percentage of therapists notifying police or documenting when a victim is specified than when one is not. Thus, for our respondents, warning the victim and notifying family or friends are relatively distinctive responses to verbal threats to harm specific persons.

13. California therapists are more likely than those practicing elsewhere to warn potential victims in response to a verbal threat identifying the victim.

Our data also show that when confronted with verbal threats and an identifiable victim, Californians warn the victim more frequently than therapists practicing in other states. About 30 percent of all warnings occur in cases not involving named victims, but these cases are equally distributed among all locations and professions. In the case of verbal threats and named victims, however, each profession in California warns at a higher rate than those located in other states. California psychiatrists are 11 percent more likely to warn potential victims than their colleagues in other jurisdictions; psychologists are five percent more likely to warn; and social workers are 20 percent more likely to warn potential victims. While differences are small for psychologists, the trend is consistent.

These results suggest that the *Tarasoff* decision has influenced behavior in those situations in which compliance seems most feasible—when a victim has been identified.

THE CONSEQUENCES OF WARNING A VICTIM

14. In general, therapists who warned potential victims in the "last dangerous case" report the same rate of subsequent attacks as those who did not.

Warning a victim appears to make virtually no difference in the incidence of attacks subsequent to actions taken to prevent potential violence. In the last dangerous case involving a patient who might harm others, 28 percent of the cases in which a warning was issued went on to attack someone subsequent to their therapists' actions; while in cases in which no warning was issued, 29 percent did so.

Subsequent attacks are most frequently reported for inpatients, and least frequently reported for private outpatients. When we take these settings into account, there are few differences in subsequent attacks by profession or location of practice.

15. Therapists who warned a victim report a lower rate of successfully resolved cases.

In slightly more than one-fourth of the cases, therapists provided us with their evaluation of the patient's condition following interventions. While therapists generally perceive their interventions as successful in that the overwhelming majority believe that the patient has improved, therapists who have warned potential victims are *less* likely than those who have not to characterize the patient as substantially improved. They are more likely to see the patient as unchanged. This difference hints at the possibility that therapists may feel that a warning takes the case "out of their hands," thus leaving the patient in roughly his or her original state.

16. Therapists commonly communicate information about patients to third parties, particularly insurers and other health professionals.

Over 80 percent of our respondents communicated information about patients to other health professionals; 70 percent to government or private health insurers; and 60 percent to a patient's family and friends in the 12 months prior to the survey. Less than 20 percent of any professional group of our respondents inside or outside of California have communicated to potential victims of their patients in the same time period.

Patient and therapist may agree about the need for the therapist to communicate with third party insurers, and little may be lost from the relationship as a result. Communications to other health professionals may stand on the same footing. Indeed, so may any communication if it is sensitively handled within the therapeutic relationship. Nonetheless, there may be communications that the therapist feels bound to make, although doing so may contradict the therapist's best clinical judgment.

17. Therapists, particularly Californians, who recently warned a potential victim are more likely than those who did not to feel that they have had to compromise their clinical judgment during their practice.

Forty-five percent of our respondents who have communicated with potential victims within a year of responding to the survey, as opposed to between 30 and 32 percent of those who have not, feel that they have had to violate their own clinical judgment in making an extra-therapeutic communication. The difference remains even when we control for the number of different extra-therapeutic communications our respondents have made. These data suggest that the therapists who warn victims are those most likely to feel that they have, at one time, acted contrary to their best clinical judgment. Warning, then, may well cut against the grain of clinical judgment for a number of our respondents.

When we break this data down by location and by profession, Californians are more likely than others to have felt compromised at some point in their careers if they have warned a potential victim. Interestingly, Californians are also more likely than others to have felt compromised at some point in their careers even if they have not warned a potential victim. While the percentage differences between Californians and others are larger in the warning situation (14 percent) than when there has been no warning (seven percent), there are far more respondents in the latter category (1,544) than in the former (144). Among the professions, psychologists are considerably less likely than either psychiatrists or social workers to feel compromised, whether or not they have ever warned a potential victim.

THE IMPACT OF *TARASOFF* ON THERAPISTS

18. Virtually all Californians, and more than one-half of those practicing elsewhere, believe themselves to be legally bound by the *Tarasoff* principle of responsibility for the physical well-being of potential victims; the clear majority of all respondents feel themselves ethically committed to this principle.

We asked our respondents who had heard of *Tarasoff* whether the principle of responsibility for the physical well-being of third parties applied to them, and why. Nine out of 10 of the California therapists believed the principle applied because *Tarasoff* was the law where they practiced. On the other hand, less than one out of five in other locations believed *Tarasoff*, or a ruling like it, applied where they practiced. However, while our respondents seem to have a fairly good understanding of the jurisdictional issue, a majority of them nonetheless believed themselves legally bound by *Tarasoff*. The primary reason for this view was the belief that the *Tarasoff* ruling applied to their professions.

Our respondents also believe that they have an ethical obligation to potential victims. With the exception of California psychiatrists, at least 60 percent of each group considers responsibility to potential victims to be a professional ethical obligation, and at least three out of four of each group consider it to be a matter of personal ethics.

Californians are considerably more likely than non-Californians to consider themselves either legally or legally and ethically bound by the *Tarasoff* principle. Those practicing outside of California are much more likely than Californians to consider themselves ethically bound only. Regardless of profession and regardless of location, only a small fraction of those who have heard of the case consider themselves neither legally nor ethically bound to protect those at risk from their patients. Indeed, there are virtually no Californians in this category, and only between 10 and 15 percent of those practicing elsewhere.

These figures certainly cast considerable doubt on the argument that *Tarasoff* offends professional ethical mandates. At the very least, our data suggest that the arguments that *Tarasoff* required deviation from ethical standards was considerably overstated or, alternatively, that the ethical standards had so tentative a hold over our respondents that within five years of the *Tarasoff* decision they have been swept aside in favor of a new *Tarasoff*-consistent ethical vision.

19. Therapists have been more willing to warn potential victims since *Tarasoff*.

We asked therapists to indicate changes between 1975 and 1980 in their willingness to employ certain interventions in the treatment of potentially violent patients. This period runs from the date of the first *Tarasoff* opinion (December, 1974) to the date of the survey, and should reflect *Tarasoff*'s influence.

Those who feel legally bound have become more willing, since *Tarasoff*, to notify potential victims (75 percent), police (48 percent), or other public authorities (59 percent) than those who believe themselves only ethically bound (60 percent, 33 percent, and 54 percent, respectively), and clearly more willing than those who don't consider themselves bound by *Tarasoff* at all (35 percent, 25 percent, and 36 percent, respectively). Ethically and legally bound therapists also are more willing to initiate involuntary hospitalization and take notes than those who feel no commitment to the *Tarasoff* principle.

Interestingly, those who view themselves as bound by *Tarasoff* do not indicate either less willingness to treat dangerous patients than the others, or more willingness to terminate treatment.

20. *Tarasoff* has not discouraged therapists from treating potentially dangerous patients.

The clear majority of all therapists have treated a dangerous patient, and a reasonably high percentage (ranging from 29 percent for "unobligated" psychologists to 60 percent for "legally bound" psychiatrists) have treated them in the past and were continuing to do so in 1980, when the survey was conducted. If the *Tarasoff* duty discourages therapists from undertaking the treatment of potentially violent patients, one would expect those who feel legally bound by *Tarasoff* to be less likely to see such patients currently. The data reveals the opposite.

Therapists who feel bound by *Tarasoff* are more likely, not less likely, than those who do not feel bound to have treated such patients during the current year and earlier. They are less likely, not more likely, to have treated such a patient prior to the current year, but not at the present time. This data on professional practices is consistent with our findings regarding changes in willingness to treat.

21. *Tarasoff* has influenced therapist action in response to the potentially violent patient, particularly in regard to warning the potential victim.

In addition to asking therapists about interventions taken in the most recent case in which they treated a patient whom they assessed as dangerous, we also asked for information about the most recent case (excluding the dangerous case) in which a patient made an explicit threat. We then selected those cases that have occurred since the *Tarasoff* decision for a further analysis of the effects of perceived legal and ethical obligation to the *Tarasoff* principle.

The results of this analysis show that therapists who believe themselves legally or ethically bound by the *Tarasoff* principle consistently warn potential victims at a higher rate than those who do not. In the dangerous case, psychiatrists who feel legally or ethically bound are 16 percent more likely to warn a victim than those who do not feel obligated by *Tarasoff*. Comparable differences for psychologists and social workers are 10 and eight points, respectively.

Furthermore, the threat case accentuates these differences. In this case, the psychiatrists who feel obligated by *Tarasoff* warn 28 percent more frequently than those who do not, while the comparable figures for psychologists and social workers are 12 percent and 17 percent, respectively.

This analysis lends further support to the conclusions drawn from an analysis of the assessment case alone. *Tarasoff* has evidently influenced therapists' behavior most markedly in situations that gave rise to the case in the first place—situations involving threatening behavior.

CONCLUSION

The *Tarasoff* decision is widely known and largely misunderstood. The misunderstandings come in two forms: a) many respondents to our survey believed the decision demanded warning when it ultimately called for reasonable care; and b) many respondents believed that they were legally bound by it when, as of the time of the survey, this was not the case (6). The decision apparently has had a significant influence on the asserted willingness of both individual therapists and institutions to notify potential victims perceived to be at risk from an imminently violent patient.

While the decision has had a marked influence on the knowledge and beliefs of therapists, we found little evidence of a dramatic, negative impact on therapeutic practice. First, most therapists do not perceive a contradiction between professional and personal ethics, on the one hand, and taking responsibility for the welfare of those threatened by patients, on the other. To the contrary, most of our respondents see this responsibility as an ethical one, in any event. While there are remaining questions of cause and effect presented by the congruence between ethical beliefs and *Tarasoff*, the very fact of this congruence suggests that *Tarasoff* did not call for a radical break with the professional mores of most of our respondents. Second, the behavior that most clearly triggers the *Tarasoff* duty—threats to identifiable individuals—is behavior that our respondents frequently identify as leading them to assess a patient as potentially violent. *Tarasoff* did not emphasize a clinically irrelevant phenomenon. Third, most therapists make communications about their patients to third parties, be they other health professionals, insurers, family, public authorities, or potential victims. *Tarasoff* did not demand unprecedented behavior. Fourth, *Tarasoff* has not led those therapists who know of it to be less willing to treat potentially violent patients or, in fact, to be less likely to have treated and to continue to treat such patients. Finally, *Tarasoff* apparently has not caused therapists to change their actions with imminently violent patients generally, except that those who know of the case and are either ethically or legally bound by it are more likely to warn potential victims. However, our respondents almost never simply warned the victim; in all but three percent of the cases in which therapists indicated that they warned a victim or recommended that this be done, they also initiated or recommended the notification of others, as well, or sought hospitalization for the patient.

The responses to our survey suggest that *Tarasoff* does not unfairly hold our respondents to nonexistent professional standards. Our respondents tended to believe that they could assess the potential for violence, and that others would agree with their assessments in a given case. Moreover, most respondents pointed to the same factors (particularly threats and violent behavior, present or current) relevant to their assessment in their most recent case.

Our study also provides little support for the view that the warning intervention, in itself, enhances public safety. The data on outcomes shows as many subsequent attacks when the warning intervention was employed or recommended as in those cases in which it was not. If anything, the outcomes data suggests that therapists who warned evaluated their interactions as slightly less successful than those who did not. Moreover, those who warned within the prior year were more likely than those who had not warned to believe that they had acted in a way that compromised their best clinical judgment at some point in their careers.

In conclusion, our data does not support the view that *Tarasoff* represents psychiatric Armageddon. Nor does it support the view that warning has proved a major boon to public safety. What *Tarasoff* has apparently done is crystallize and shape beliefs concerning a therapist's obligation to protect those at risk from a patient. It has also influenced therapist attitudes and practices regarding notifying those to whom the patient represents a threat. It is unfortunate that the decision has been understood so narrowly, since there are surely situations in which the false belief that a therapist must warn will prove counterproductive to working with the patient, or protecting the victim, or both. However, some therapists have worked successfully with the warning intervention (7), and, no doubt, even more could do so if the case comes to be viewed as asking therapists to exercise care and judgment in dealing with the potentially violent patient.

References

1. As we make clear in the text, there were two decisions. The final and *official* opinion is *Tarasoff v. Board of Regents of University of California* 17 Cal. 3rd 425, 551 P. 2d 334, 131 Cal. Rptr. 14 (1976).

The initial decision, now withdrawn, appeared, under the same name, in 13 Cal. 3rd 177, 529 P., 2d 553, 118 Cal. Rptr. 129 (1974).

2. These criticisms, and others, are developed in Stone AA: The *Tarasoff* decision: suing psychotherapists to safeguard security. Harvard Law Review 90: 358–378, 1976; Gurevitz, H: *Tarasoff*: protective privilege versus public peril. Am J Psychiatry 134: 289–292, 1977; Roth L, Meisel A: Dangerousness, confidentiality and the duty to warn. Am J Psychiatry 134: 508–511, 197.

3. Wise TP: Where the public peril begins: a survey of psychotherapists to determine the effects of *Tarasoff*. Stanford Law Review 31:165–190, 1978.

4. For a fuller report of the methodology and survey instrument, consult Givelber D, Bowers W, Blitch C: *Tarasoff*, myth and reality: an empirical study. Wisconsin Law Review (2); 443–497, 1984.

5. The data referred to in this paper are presented in a more complete form in the Myth and Reality paper, n.3 *supra*, and two working papers of the Center for Applied Social Research, Northeastern University, Boston, Mass.: Bowers W, Givelber D, Blitch C: Do judicial decisions affect clinical practice?; and Blitch C, Bowers W, Givelber D: Assessing dangerousness: criteria cited by mental health professionals.

6. As of the mailing of the survey in spring 1980, the only court which had applied *Tarasoff* to a psychiatrist's failure to protect an identifiable victim from a potentially violent patient was the New Jersey Superior Court in *McIntosh v. Milano*, 168 N.J. Super. 466, 403 A. 2d 500 (1979). Since that time a number of Courts have cited and ruled on *Tarasoff* but, as of the spring of 1984, only a few other State Supreme Courts have officially embraced *Tarasoff*. See Myth and Reality, n.3 *supra*, for a brief review of the decisions.

7. For example, see Beck JC: When the patient threatens violence: an empirical study of clinical practice after *Tarasoff*. Bulletin of the American Academy of Psychiatry and Law 10:189–201, 1982; Roth L, Meisel A: n.2 *supra*; Wulsin LR, Bursztajn J, Gutheil TG: Unexpected clinical features of the *Tarasoff* decision: the therapeutic alliance and the duty to warn. Am J Psychiatry 140:601–603, 1983.

4

A Clinical Survey of the *Tarasoff* Experience

James C. Beck, M.D., Ph.D.

4

A Clinical Survey of the *Tarasoff* Experience

Commentators on the clinical implications of the *Tarasoff* duty have not been in agreement. Stone (1) suggested that the *Tarasoff* duty would lead to more danger, not less, since potential patients would be deterred from entering therapy by the threat to their confidentiality. He thought that this would be an especially difficult problem for clients whose problems included drug abuse, or involvement with the criminal justice system. By contrast, Slovenko noted that, "trust—not absolute confidentiality—is the cornerstone of psychotherapy. Talking about a patient or writing about him without his knowledge or consent would be a breach of trust. But imposing control where self-control breaks down is not a breach of trust when it is not deceptive (2)." Wechsler argued that the *Tarasoff* duty was best discharged by bringing the potential victim and the patient together in a conjoint therapy in which the therapist attempted to help the two deal with their situation without recourse to violence (3).

There have been few published *Tarasoff* cases. Roth and Meisel reported four cases from an emergency room, only one of which involved a warning (4). They believe so strongly in the importance of informed consent that they have always discussed the proposed action with the patient. Wulsin et al. (5) describe a case from an inpatient service in which the patient's threats to kill his mother were of sufficient concern that the staff felt obligated to inform her of them. They discussed their concerns extensively with the patient and they planned jointly with him to warn his mother. He and his mother had a tearful conversation in which they told each other that they loved each other, and no violence ensued. The authors concluded that their efforts to meet the *Tarasoff* duty had been beneficial to the patient and had strengthened the therapeutic alliance.

This chapter presents cases I have collected from two sources: colleagues of mine and psychiatrists in private practice outside of major cities, who were not affiliated with academic departments of psychiatry. I chose to collect these latter cases because of Gurevitz's observation that practitioners appeared to see grave problems with the *Tarasoff* duty, where academic psychiatrists did not. The remainder of this chapter presents these cases along with brief comments.

Case Example 1

A single male graduate student became delusional, unable to work, and seclusive. He was hospitalized and treated with phenothiazines and individual psychotherapy by Dr. A, a resident. Coincidentally, a lifelong friend of the patient was also treated by Dr. A, and this friend committed suicide.

The patient was discharged and was to be followed up by Dr. A, but terminated treatment six weeks later in a dispute over medication. After an intervening commitment to a state hospital, the patient reappeared at the outpatient department where he said that he was thinking of killing Dr. A. Outpatient staff consulted Dr. Z, a staff psychiatrist. Dr. Z interviewed the patient and offered him treatment, which he accepted.

The patient said Dr. A had killed some of his brain cells by prescribing a poisonous drug, Thorazine, and he held Dr. A responsible for the suicide of his friend. He repeatedly said that he would like to kill Dr. A. He recalled that he had won a rifle medal as an adolescent, and said he was still an excellent shot. He did not own a gun, and there was no history of violence.

The patient's anger at Dr. A persisted. A chance meeting with Dr. A would stimulate the patient to murderous ideation. Dr. Z never believed that the patient was imminently murderous, but he thought the patient might impulsively assault Dr. A.

Dr. Z decided a warning was necessary. He first discussed this with the patient, saying he was concerned for the safety of Dr. A and for the welfare of the patient, and wished to protect them both. The patient agreed that Dr. Z should speak with Dr. A, and Dr. Z subsequently did so. Dr. A, who lived near the patient and who had previously met the patient by chance several times on the street, was grateful for the warning, and took action to avoid meeting the patient thereafter.

Psychotherapy continued for several years. Dr. Z made repeated efforts to explore possible deeper danger meanings of the patient's hostility to Dr. A. Recall of memories of parental neglect and of the patient's subsequent anger and disappointment seemed to relate to the patient's concerns about whether Dr. Z was trustworthy. Recall of a childhood relationship with a neighborhood physician clarified the basis for some of the patient's positive feelings toward Dr. Z, but no attempt to understand the affect and dynamics produced any change in the patient's sense of having been betrayed by Dr. A.

The patient consistently refused medicine. At termination, he was living independently, had some friends, held a full-time professional job, was free of delusional beliefs concerning his current life, but was still angry at Dr. A.

One year later Dr. Z asked the patient, "Do you remember whether my warning Dr. A made any difference one way or the other in therapy?"

The patient responded, "I have a vivid memory. I respected your response. I thought, 'that was a very wise response. I've just been really bizarre here. What would I have done sitting in his place?' It's amazing to me that you asked me. If there is one psychological barrier I have not overcome, it's Dr. A. I fantasize about killing Dr. A and about Dr. A's death. The only thing that prevents me is prison . . . "

Dr. Z expressed concern about the patient's continued wish to kill Dr. A. The patient responded that Dr. Z did not need to worry on his account.

Over the next three years the patient consulted Dr. Z on several occasions. He continued to work effectively in his new career, and he established an enduring intimate heterosexual relationship. Eventually, he decided to return to graduate school and devote himself to the work he liked best, using his professional skills to support his intellectual pursuits. To this end, he moved 1,000 miles away. Several years earlier, Dr. A moved 2,000 miles in another direction.

Comment: In this case the warning was clinically indicated, and it was discussed with the patient as a therapeutic issue rather than as a realistic constraint imposed on the therapist. The impact of the discussion of the possible danger and the need to take action appeared to have a positive effect on the development of the therapeutic alliance at the time, and as reported a year later by the patient.

In this case, warning was indicated and commitment was not. Dr. Z never believed the patient was imminently murderous or that the danger of impulsive assault was sufficiently likely to justify involuntary hospitalization. The patient had no history of violence, owned no gun, and did have a therapeutic alliance.

The warning may have helped prevent violence in that it permitted Dr. A to successfully avoid chance meetings with the patient, meetings which had previously provoked the patient's murderous fantasies. Certainly, Dr. A was glad to have been warned and believed that he was able to use the warning to change his behavior constructively. The long-term follow-up of the patient and Dr. A permits the conclusion that the danger of violence had passed.

Case Example 2

A depressed, somewhat phobic grandmother was in group therapy in an outpatient clinic. In group she had mentioned, but without much intensity, some fear that she might harm her infant grandson, whom she cared for regularly. During a medication consulation with the therapist's supervisor and the therapist, the patient said with considerable intensity that she was afraid she might strangle the infant. The patient was frightened by these thoughts. The supervisor told the patient and the therapist that the therapist should inform the patient's daughter of the threat to her son.

The patient again discussed her fears in the group, and then the therapist met with her individually. The therapist shared with the patient her own worry that the patient had to live with so much anxiety about the baby, and her concern that there was some risk that it might really happen. She told the patient that, as a professional, she had a legal responsibility to inform the mother of the baby, but that for now the therapist wanted only to talk it over with the patient.

The patient was furious with the supervisor, both for his style and for what he said. She resented his apparent conviction that she might actually strangle the baby, and she resented that he had not given her the opportunity to explore her feelings more fully. As she talked with the therapist she became extremely anxious, and the therapist told her they could handle it together. They agreed on a plan in which the therapist would call the mother in the patient's presence, explain the problem, and then put the patient on the phone to talk to her daughter. The therapist made the call and focused on whether the daughter was aware of how much stress the baby-sitting was placing on the patient. The daughter was understanding, and reacted to her mother in a supportive way. The frequency of baby-sitting was subsequently reduced, and the patient discussed the entire episode in the group. The therapist believed that the alliance was strengthened by sharing this experience.

Comment: This is an example of a case in which the warning was discussed extensively and integrated into the therapeutic experience. The therapist thought that the alliance had been strengthened as a result, and there was a good practical resolution to the problem, as well.

Case Example 3

A married woman in her 40s had a long history of stormy personal relationships. She had many depersonalization experiences in which she would bite her own arms. She had made strangling motions as well during some of these episodes. Her husband filed for divorce, and she then cut her wrists and threatened suicide. She was admitted voluntarily to a psychiatric ward where she confided in her physician that she planned to kill her husband using either a knife, a gun, or poison, but she refused to say when this might occur. Her physician consulted the ward administrator, who consulted the hospital administration, who consulted the hospital lawyer, who advised warning the husband. The physician sent the husband a letter of warning and then told the patient and the hospital administration that she had done so. The hospital lawyer was furious because the letter had not been sent by registered mail. The patient was furious and refused to talk with her physician for two weeks. When a therapeutic dialogue was re-established, the patient spent several hours talking about how betrayed and angry she felt. At discharge six weeks later, the patient acknowledged that she recognized that the doctor had acted correctly. The patient returned to her outpatient therapist. Eighteen months later she killed herself.

Comment: The effect of warning with and without discussion can be clearly distinguished. The warning was given without prior discussion and it had an immediate negative impact on the therapeutic relationship; the patient felt angry and betrayed. The therapist realized that she had been responding to the adminstrative–legal concerns raised by her superiors, and that she had acted without thinking carefully about the possible effect on the patient. Later, the physician understood and accepted the patient's wrath, and encouraged the patient to share these feelings. The patient's anger then subsided, and she was able to acknowledge that the therapist had acted reasonably.

It is clear that this patient possessed a potential for violent action. Perhaps the warning served a limit-setting function that helped the patient control her potentially violent impulses over

the impending divorce. Nothing is known about the circumstances of the later suicide.

Case Example 4

A single man in his 20s with a diagnosis of chronic schizophrenia was treated by a psychiatrist in a community mental health
clinic. The patient believed a local university was trying to drive
him crazy by planting in the minds of little girls that he was a notorious masturbator. He would often call the university to make
bomb threats. In the psychiatrist's office he talked about killing
young women, one in particular, but he did not identify her or
know where she lived. He broke all the windows in the office, and
had thrown plants and a jar of honey against the wall. Neither oral
antipsychotic medication nor psychotherapy had any effect on
this patient. There was never a specific victim to warn, but the
psychiatrist had seriously considered warning the university.

On several occasions, the patient had threatened to commit
suicide by immolating himself with gasoline in his sleeping bag.
The psychiatrist told the patient he had a duty to intervene to
protect the patient, and possibly to warn the landlady. On two
occasions, the patient was involuntarily hospitalized. Neither the
possibility of warning the landlady nor the actuality of commitment appeared to have any long-term effect on this patient. After
each hospitalization the patient returned to the psychiatrist for
follow-up treatment, chronically psychotic but not acutely disturbed. Finally, the patient was given intramuscular Prolixin with
dramatic improvement. On four-year follow-up the patient was
no longer actively psychotic, and had re-established social relationships with his family and some of his old acquaintances. He told
the psychiatrist it must have been awful for him to be with the patient while he was so ill, and he apologized for his past behavior in
the office.

Comment: There is no evidence that the psychiatrist's attempts
to treat this patient effectively and to prevent violence by involuntary hospitalization interfered with the eventual successful treatment of this patient. The psychiatrist always discussed his con-

cerns with the patient before committing him, or when considering warning the landlady, and the patient always returned for treatment when he had free choice as to whether to return or not. When he was finally treated with an effective psychopharmacologic regimen, he demonstrated, by his apology, that he was personally concerned about the psychiatrist.

Commitment rather than warning was indicated because the patient was mentally ill with a history of violence. He had the means to carry out his threatened immolation, and there was a shaky therapeutic alliance. Once committed there was no need to warn the landlady because the danger no longer existed. The psychiatrist considered warning the university but never did so, because he never considered that the bomb threats constituted a real danger. They were always made in association with the patients delusional fantasies, and the patient did not know how to make a bomb, had no access to explosives, and had no plan for any realistic accomplishment of this fantasied threat. Although we cannot say with certainty that treatment prevented violence, treatment was eventually successful, and the patient was never violent outside the psychiatrist's office as far as is known.

This is an example of a case in which warning and commitment were discussed ahead of time. There appeared to be no discernable effect on the treatment resulting from the possible warning and the actual commitment.

Case Example 5

A college student who was severely disabled by a congenital abnormality and a borderline personality disorder was being treated in psychoanalysis. He had a profoundly ambivalent relationship with his mother, and he owned an axe that he kept sharpened. He expressed fantasies of beheading an anonymous woman and raping her. The analyst discussed the question of thought versus action in the analytic situation, and told the patient that any such action would harm him as well as the victim. Eventually, the roots of the fantasy were analyzed, and the patient got rid of the axe. The analyst never found it necessary to breach the patient's confidentiality or involve any third person.

Comment: In this case, the analyst thought that the possibility of action was remote because there was no history of violence, no history of loss of emotional control, and there was a reasonably good therapeutic alliance. Therefore, the analyst concluded that no action was immediately necessary, and he felt ultimately that this decision was correct after the additional therapeutic work had been done.

Case Example 6

A mother of two, separated and in her mid-30s had been repeatedly and unsuccessfully treated by a community mental health center. She presented at the emergency service stating that she had set several fires and was thinking of setting more. In the past, the patient had made dramatic threats and/or claims; for example that she was suffocating in a phone booth, or that she had set a major fire. She had slashed her wrists once, and was believed to have set two fires—one in a treatment facility, and one in a former therapist's car.

The evaluating psychiatrist believed she was potentially dangerous, and he offered her a choice: either she would agree to outpatient treatment and the psychiatrist would notify the fire marshall, or she could be hospitalized at the state hospital. She chose outpatient treatment, and the psychiatrist notified the fire marshall. The patient was followed for several years thereafter. She set no further fires in the mental health system, nor did she make any new threats to mental health center staff.

Comment: Firm limits, including a warning to appropriate authorities, were set as an initial condition for treatment of this difficult and potentially violent patient. We do not know whether the patient improved. We do know that she did not engage in the kind of troublesome behavior that had marked her history.

Case Example 7

A single 23-year-old factory worker planted a bomb at his work place and then told the authorities what he had done. Clinical diagnosis was psychosis and schizoid character. An independent psychiatrist reviewing the case diagnosed schizoid character with antisocial traits.

The patient was tried and convicted, and given a suspended sentence with one year of psychiatric treatment as a condition of probation. The patient attended individual psychotherapy sessions weekly, as prescribed, but his therapist believed that no alliance had been established and that the patient remained aloof, distant, and essentially uninvolved. In therapy the patient expressed rage at his parents, and no regrets for what he had done. When his probation status ended, he abruptly terminated therapy. Reviewing the case after the patient terminated, the therapist and his supervisor both believed that the patient was potentially dangerous to his parents. The Court and the parents were so advised, and the patient was notified in writing of the therapist's decision. Two years later, while the parents were sleeping, he assaulted them with a heavy club. He broke their arms and legs and scarred the face of one.

Comment: There is not good evidence that this patient had a treatable mental disorder. He had no apparent motivation to examine his own character or his violent impulses. No alliance was established. Whether psychiatric treatment is preferable to probationary supervision is questionable. In similar cases assigned to our Court clinic, we have tried psychiatric supervision rather than more traditional psychotherapy. Supervision appears better suited to the needs of these patients and society than is more traditional psychotherapy.

In this case, the warning was not discussed with the patient, because the need for action only emerged after the patient terminated. This is an example of a case in which the warning was not discussed, and ultimately violence occurred: a very bad outcome, indeed. Whether the outcome would have been different if the patient had been called back in for a prior consultation is speculative. Similarly, whether it would have been helpful to the parents in dealing with their son to have called them in for a conference, rather than writing to them, is an open question. Wechsler would suggest that the most appropriate therapeutic intervention in a case of this nature would be to bring the parents and the son in for joint psychotherapy sessions, in which the issues of rage and potential violence are openly discussed (3).

Would commitment have been preferable to warning? The therapist considered commitment and discussed it with his supervisor, but they rejected this alternative on two grounds: first, there was no good evidence of psychosis—the patient was neither delusional nor hallucinating, and his thought was not grossly disordered; second, there was no evidence of imminent danger—the patient was not threatening anyone, and indeed he was not violent until two years later.

Case Example 8

A single man in his late 20s with a diagnosis of chronic schizoaffective disorder, was treated in private outpatient psychotherapy. The patient threatened to kill his parents, with whom he lived. When interviewed some time later, the psychiatrist stated that he had informed the patient that it was necessary to warn the parents, and after discussing the warning with the patient, he had warned the parents. The patient became acutely agitated and grossly psychotic shortly thereafter, and required hospitalization.

The hospital physician reported that the patient was furious at his private psychiatrist, and actively psychotic. The patient said that his private psychiatrist had not told him about his proposed breach of confidentiality. The patient remained in the hospital for months, psychotic and unable to progress. In the opinion of the hospital physician, the angry impasse resulted from the patient's sense of betrayal by the therapist.

Comment: This case illustrates a warning associated with a bad outcome. What the therapist actually said is unclear; what is clear is that the patient experienced the warning as unexpected, felt betrayed, and was subsequently chronically psychotic and severely impaired.

Case Example 9

A depressed 23-year-old woman was treated in a psychiatric hospital. She told her psychiatrist she might throw her baby against the wall. He was convinced she might carry out this threat, and he told her in a ward meeting that he had no option but to protect the child. He presented this to her as a fixed decision over which she had no control, and he then informed the appropriate social agency. The patient became increasingly anxious and depressed. Later, the patient and her psychiatrist discussed her feelings. She told him, "I could understand why you did it, but it would have helped if you had discussed it with me." The psychiatrist commented, "I was so anxious about it I didn't discuss it enough with the patient. Afterward, when we had talked, she felt better about it. If I had another case like it, I would give the patient the opportunity to discuss it beforehand."

Case Example 10

A 28-year-old white male, who was separated, was referred to an emergency service for evaluation by his lawyer. The history as it emerged from the patient, his lawyer, and eventually the police, was that the patient had beaten his wife repeatedly, and she had taken their young children and left him. He then became convinced that she was "sleeping around" and he was suspicious that his best friend was one of her lovers.

He went to his lawyer's office carrying a loaded gun, told the lawyer he was planning to shoot and kill his wife and his friend, and asked what the penalty would be. The lawyer relieved the patient of his gun, advised him that it would be big trouble if he carried out his threat, brought the patient to the emergency room, and then gave the gun to the police.

The patient was a Vietnam veteran who owned a large gun and ammunition collection, including a machine gun. He was a karate expert with a history of many fights. He was suspected of being a drug dealer, and he associated with gangsters. He had been in an auto accident, and sustained brain damage that prevented him from working regularly.

The psychiatrist believed he was dealing with a man who had an acute marital problem, an organic brain syndrome, probable antisocial personality, and drug and alcohol abuse. He was impressed with how much pain the patient was feeling because of the separation from his wife and children. He told the patient that this must be driving him crazy, and the patient acknowledged that it was. The patient said, furthermore, that his friends were taunting him to kill his wife and his friend, saying that he wasn't a man unless he did. The patient wanted to leave town to get away from the pressure he felt, but told the psychiatrist he was unable to do so for reasons he would not disclose.

The psychiatrist told the patient that he was not crazy and certainly would be held responsible for any violent act, and he urged the patient to return to the emergency service for further treatment. He also told the patient that he would tell the police and his lawyer that he was threatening his wife and friend. There was no way to warn the wife directly, as neither the patient nor the lawyer knew where she was. The patient was furious, mostly at his lawyer, when he found out that the lawyer had turned the gun over to the police. When the psychiatrist called the police he found that the patient was well known to them, because of his participation in gang fights and other violent and criminal activities.

The patient returned several times to see the psychiatrist. While checking throughout the mental health center, the psychiatrist found that the wife was in treatment in a satellite clinic. Subsequently the wife's therapist suggested that the patient attend the wife's therapy sessions for some couples work. Several appointments were scheduled but the patient missed them all. Over a period of several weeks the patient's rage gradually subsided, and he gradually gave up the idea of killing his wife and friend. However, he began drinking heavily, and was referred to the alcoholism service. Ultimately, he moved out of the catchment area and was referred to the facility serving his new locale.

Comment: This is a warning that is typical of emergency room *Tarasoff* interventions. The police already knew a great deal more about the patient and his activities than the mental health system knew, and the warning probably was of trivial practical significance. As far as was known, the patient was not violent during the period he was treated by this facility. The warning was discussed ahead of time with the patient, and although it made him angry, by his own report other actions made him angrier, and he was not driven out of treatment by his anger.

Case Example 11

A schizophrenic woman seen in a private office threatened to kill her husband. The patient had often been angry at the husband, but had never seriously assaulted him. The patient's husband frequently telephoned the psychiatrist to discuss his wife's condition. In the course of one of these conversations, the psychiatrist reported the threat to the husband. The husband did not believe that he was in any serious danger, and did not think any action was required. The psychiatrist never told the patient he was talking with her husband, because he feared it might alienate her. The patient eventually stopped taking her medicine, made a serious suicide attempt, and was committed to the state hospital.

Comment: This is an example of a case in which the warning was not discussed with the patient as a therapeutic issue, and there was a bad outcome.

Case Example 12

A borderline woman seen in a private office had seriously assaulted her children. Under the law, the psychiatrist was required to notify the State Children's Service Agency when he became aware that the children were at risk of harm from their mother. The psychiatrist spent two sessions discussing with the patient the fact that he was required to report this to the authorities, and discussing with her its potential usefulness to her and the children. The patient consented to notification of the authorities. Sometime later the patient terminated, partly for financial reasons, and partly because she was unhappy about his having reported the child abuse. After the appropriate investigation, her children remained with her, and subsequently they assaulted her with a deadly weapon.

Comment: The warning did not serve to prevent violence, and had some negative impact on the psychotherapy. It is difficult, however, to suggest a better course of action, since the psychiatrist was required by law to notify the social agency, and he acted correctly in doing so.

Case Example 13

A married man in his 40s, seen in a private office, had a history of impulsive violence and had assaulted his children. Although the patient's wife was aware of the patient's history, she minimized any possible current threat to herself or the children. The psychiatrist believed that both she and the children were at risk of being assaulted, and he told the patient that it was necessary to bring his wife into the office for a discussion. The patient agreed. The psychiatrist discussed the child abuse with her in the patient's presence.

The psychiatrist commented, "It was enormously helpful to psychotherapy. It got the wife to take him more seriously. She took seriously the things he was pleading for. Before he would yell at her and ask for answers and she would be silent, absolutely silent, and he got more furious. That changed." On six month follow-up there had been no further violence.

Comment: This is an example of a case in which the need for a warning was discussed as part of the therapy, the patient's consent was obtained, and the potential victim was brought into the psychotherapeutic situation so that the warning itself became part of the therapy. The effect on the therapy and on the marriage appeared to be positive.

Case Example 14

A man in his 60s, suffering from a chronic depressive disorder, was in private psychotherapy. His psychiatrist was away, and he was seen by a colleague of his therapist. During the session the patient said that a former colleague of his "did not have the right to live." He also said that he was planning to withdraw some money from the bank, and visit the community in which the former colleague lived. Although the patient seemed to be in good control and had no known history of violence, the psychiatrist was concerned and reported the threat to the local police without discussing this with the patient.

When the treating psychiatrist returned and heard the story, he was sufficiently impressed with the potential for violence that he asked the local police to pick the patient up and bring him to the emergency room, which they did. The patient denied any violent intent, and made light of the whole episode in a way that the psychiatrist found entirely convincing.

The psychiatrist told me that he spent some months thereafter going over this episode in therapy, focusing especially on how the patient was the person principally responsible for what had occurred. The psychiatrist thought that the therapeutic discussion had been useful to the patient, and that the case had gone well.

Comment: This is a case in which the warning was not discussed ahead of time with the patient, and in which the patient was apprehended by the police. There was a good therapeutic relationship, and the therapist focused on the clinical implications of the patient's behavior rather than on the possible legal consequences to himself. The psychiatrist thought he had been able to use the episode positively to further the patient's understanding of how he created his own difficulties. Perhaps the moral is *coniunctio bona omnia vincit:* a good alliance conquers all.

Case Example 15

A psychiatrist working in a private psychiatric hospital admitted a divorced white male in his 20s who was drug dependent and had a mixed personality disorder. The patient said his ex-wife had had an affair before they were separated, and that she was currently dating someone. He was jealous and angry, and he had threatened her with assault. During the admission conference, he told the psychiatrist that he had also threatened his ex-wife's boyfriend to his face, and he said, "I'm going to kill him." The psychiatrist told the patient that she had a duty to warn the potential victim. The patient left the hospital against medical advice immediately after the conference. The psychiatrist warned the ex-wife, who in turn warned the boyfriend. The psychiatrist commented that she did not feel much pressure to warn in this case, because the wife already knew her ex-husband was threatening.

Comment: This is an example of the chilling effect on patients that Stone predicted would result from *Tarasoff* (1). The psychiatrist, who worked full-time in the private hospital, estimated that she warned four or five potential victims a year, and that in two of these cases the patient left the hospital as a result.

Case Example 16

A single white man in his mid-20s came voluntarily to an outpatient clinic. Evaluation revealed that he was charged with armed robbery and that he thought his case might be helped if he were in treatment. He claimed to be innocent, and he alleged that he was standing on a street corner when the armed robber ran past him and thrust the gun into his hands. The police, who were chasing the robber, came along a moment later and arrested him.

As an adolescent he had been treated for four years in a psychoanalytically oriented psychiatric hospital. Currently, he was on Social Security disability, and living with 10 to 12 people in a squalid apartment. Some of his roommates were chronically drunk and often screamed late at night. He described himself as politically conscious, spending much of his time demonstrating on behalf of the oppressed.

He did not seem particularly depressed or elated. His thought was clear and connected; there was no evidence of delusions or hallucinations. He was troubled about his future, and had been in jail enough so that he knew that two or three years in prison would not be pleasant. He was offered, and accepted, membership in a group whose purpose was to provide immediate treatment for persons who appeared to be in acute distress, and for whom no other disposition was available. He was told that this group would be used in his case for an extended evaluation of how, if at all, the clinic could be useful to him.

He attended the group regularly in spite of the fact that the leader announced that he would be leaving after 12 sessions. After four sessions he came in looking forlorn and said in a muted voice that he had been "really suicidal." The leader asked him what he meant. The patient said, "You know, man, I've been planning."

The therapist said again that he did not understand what the patient meant and so he needed to ask again. The patient said again that he was suicidal and that the therapist knew what he meant, or should know if he were any good. He then embarked on a monologue about the lousy world, the downtrodden, neglected, oppressed souls, street people, and women who might get raped.

The therapist redirected the patient's attention to the thoughts of suicide, saying he thought they were fantasies. The patient said they were not fantasies, and that this showed the psychiatrist did not understand him. He returned to the subject of what a lousy world it is, and he offered the psychiatrist to the group as an example of how lousy the world is. Again, the therapist asked what exactly were the suicidal plans. The patient said that he would grab a police officer's gun during the upcoming trial and shoot the police officer, and that he himself would then be shot and killed. Alternately, he talked about going into a "cop shop," and grabbing a gun from a police officer and shooting him, and again being killed himself.

The therapist said this was a fantasy about hurting other people. The patient replied, "If you think that's a fantasy, you don't understand people. That's a plan." The therapist said again that the patient talked about being suicidal, but the plan is one to hurt other people. The patient said, "What do you think will happen when I do that?" He then added a statement about hating the police, having nothing to live for, being angry about what's ahead (that is, his trial), and he might as well finish it this way, or take them with him.

The group failed to respond to any of this, and talked about other matters for 10 minutes. The therapist then returned to the patient's plans and stated his *Tarasoff* responsibilities. He said that he had an obligation to try to protect the patient and others from potential violence, adding that he did not think the patient was mentally ill (therefore commitment was not indicated), and that he was not sure what else he could do. The therapist conveyed his concern that the patient not hurt himself or others.

The patient said, "I thought everything I said was confidential." The therapist said that was so unless there was a threat of violence. The therapist pointed out that the patient knew that the therapist had the power to commit him and that this involved a breach of confidentiality.

The patient said, "I'm not 100 percent sure it's the right thing to do," (that is, to shoot a police officer). "It's something I'm thinking about. I came here looking for help. You don't think I'm mentally ill?"

"No, I don't," the therapist answered.

"What do you think?"

"I think you're a troubled person, angry and scared."

The patient then again attacked the therapist—"Shrinks don't do any good, you don't understand people. You're no good." The therapist went on to talk about how he thought it had been a great struggle for the patient to get where he was in life, and that he had to fight against feelings of worthlessness and hopelessness and suicidal thoughts for many years.

The patient acknowledged that his life had been a struggle, and that at least some part of him was hopeful that life could improve. The therapist said that sometimes, when people get older, they can handle their problems better.

The patient said that he hoped this was so, and because of this hope he questioned whether he would want to endanger his life as well as the lives of innocent people, the police, or Court officers, in a shootout. The patient then asked more directly for help. He said that he had recently tried to contact his former psychiatrist, and that he needed more help than a once-a-week group; he needed a program, and he did not want to go to the state hospital.

The therapist then talked about leaving the group, and how this patient and others might feel that they were not getting enough, and would miss the therapist. He suggested a concrete plan for referring this patient to a day-treatment program.

Comment: A co-therapist/trainee wrote, "The therapist probes the question of suicide and the patient's 'plan' many times before the 'plan' is actually revealed. The therapist is persistent and constantly refers back to quizzing the patient as to what he intends to do. While the therapist is persistent, he allows the patient to express himself. The persistence, staying with the patient, somehow solidified the relationship. Eventually, the neediness of the patient is revealed. Trust between the two is reinforced when the issue of confidentiality is raised, and both are able to and do state their positions. The therapist acknowledges the patient's neediness as well as how he will miss the therapist."

In later group sessions the patient repeatedly voiced the concern that he would not get a fair trial ("it's a lousy world"), and that he would be convicted in spite of his innocence, which he consistently maintained ("I am one of the oppressed"). He dropped out after a few weeks, but was never violent as far as is known. He defaulted on his Court appearance, and we believe he left the state.

Case Examples 17 and 18

In the survey of private practitioners there were two instances in which a psychiatrist reported that he was the potential victim of another therapist's patient. In each case, the therapist had warned the psychiatrist of possible danger. In one case, the clinic in which a psychiatrist worked notified him that an ex-patient of his had threatened to kill him. The psychiatrist commented, "The effect of the warning was to make me a little more cautious and not take chances. I parked my car a little further away from the office than usual. I thought about whether the guy could reach me or not, and I concluded that he could not. I was not terribly fearful. The warning was helpful to me. I conferred with the crisis service and got a sense of what they were going to do, and what they thought I should do. They saw the patient a few times, and he calmed down."

In the other case, a psychiatrist had previously committed a patient who had since been discharged and was currently in treatment with another therapist. The patient had a history of making bomb threats, but had never carried out such a threat. The patient told his therapist that he planned to bomb the psychiatrist's house. The therapist reported the threat to the psychiatrist, but said she would do nothing further. She told the patient she would see him in three weeks. The psychiatrist was severely distressed and tried to press criminal charges but could not because the threat had not been made to him. He told me, *"Tarasoff* is just crazy. It specifically applies to why I carry mace. There's not a goddam thing I can do unless the therapist is willing to come in and testify. The poor potential victim has no recourse."

Comment: These two cases in which the psychiatrist was threatened illustrate the importance of responsible action by the therapist. In the first case, the clinic team dealt effectively with the patient, and the potential victim dealt constructively with the threat. In the second case, the therapist's failure to stay in close and frequent contact with the patient, and her refusal to involve the criminal justice system, led to a sense of vulnerability in the potential victim—a sense that persisted and generalized beyond the original situation.

CONCLUSION

The principal regularity to be discerned among these cases is a clear relationship between the way in which the warning is given and its impact on the psychotherapy. Cases in which the clinician discusses the warning with the patient before giving it typically show no bad effects resulting from the warning. In some of these cases, especially when the therapist clearly sees the potential violence as a therapeutic issue (and correspondingly sees the duty to warn as having clinical relevance), the discussion of the warning appears to have a positive impact on the psychotherapeutic process, and on the development of the alliance. Conversely, the cases in which the warning is not discussed ahead of time often turn out badly, and it is clear from the patient reports that patients resent warnings that are given without their knowledge.

The effectiveness of these warnings in preventing violence is difficult to assess. The observations of the resident in Case Example 1 and of the two psychiatrists in Cases Examples 16 and

17 are unique in giving us the victim's perspective. The effect of the warning clearly depends upon the circumstances of the particular case, and on how the therapist of the potentially violent patient behaves. When victims think that they can take effective evasive action, and when they are confident that the treating professionals are acting constructively and providing them with the information they need to protect themselves, they feel that the warnings have a positive effect. In sharp contrast, when victims see no possible course of evasive action and when they think that the therapist is not behaving responsibly the warning has a profoundly negative impact. As with the patient, so with the victim: how the warning is given, not whether one is given, is the crucial factor determining the impact of the warning.

References

1. Stone A: The *Tarasoff* decisions: suing psychotherapists to safeguard society. Harvard Law Review 90:358-370, 1976

2. Slovenko R: Psychotherapy and confidentiality. Clev St. L Rev 24:375-391, 1975

3. Wechsler DB: Patients, therapists and third parties: the victimological virtues of *Tarasoff*. International Journal of Law and Psychiatry 2:1-28, 1979

4. Roth LH, Meisel A: Dangerousness, confidentiality, and the duty to warn. Am J Psychiatry 134:508-511, 1977

5. Wulsin LR, et al: Unexpected clinical features of the *Tarasoff* decision: the therapeutic alliance and the "duty to warn". Am J Psychiatry 140:601-603, 1983

6. Gurevitz H: *Tarasoff*: protective privilege versus public peril. Am J Psychiatry 134:289-292, 1977

Psychiatric Assessment of Potential Violence: A Reanalysis of the Problem

James C. Beck, M.D., Ph.D.

5

Psychiatric Assessment of Potential Violence: A Reanalysis of the Problem

The psychiatric assessment of the potentially violent patient confronts us with an apparent contradiction. Study after study (such as 1, 2) show that psychiatrists are unable to predict violence with sufficient accuracy to be useful in the individual case. This fact is now generally known, and is often quoted not only in professional writing, but in public remarks by eminent psychiatrists. Judges and others in the legal profession also know it well. Yet, in spite of this knowledge, psychiatrists continue to believe that they can predict violence. As we saw in Chapter Three of this monograph, over 75 percent of psychiatrists said they could predict, "probably or certainly," whether or not an outpatient they were treating would harm someone. Moreover, 70 percent believed that 90 to 100 percent of their colleagues would agree with their predictions.

Society continues to demand that psychiatrists predict violence. A prerequisite for involuntary commitment in most states is a statement by a psychiatrist or other qualified physician that failure to hospitalize would create a likelihood of serious harm by reason of mental illness, either to the patient or to someone else. This language is nothing more or less than a requirement that psychiatrists make judgments of committability based on a prediction of potential future violence.

It is unusual for a belief to persist in the face of scientific evidence that contradicts it. As psychiatrists concerned with understanding the irrational and its basis in human experience, we have some expertise that may help us to understand this phenomenon. Since the understanding of it has important implications for clinical practice, it is essential to our professional well-being that we try.

Although psychiatrists know in an abstract way that there is no evidence that they can predict violence, almost none of us understands why this should be so. Many, and, I suspect, most psychiatrists, myself included, believe they can predict violence even if the profession as a whole apparently cannot. One common argument that purports to explain the inaccuracy of psychiatrists' predictions is that psychiatrists conservatively over-predict violence, because the consequences of over-prediction are more benign than those of under-prediction. Thus, the psychiatrist who believes that he or she would not over-predict has a substantive basis for believing that he or she would more accurately predict violence than would other psychiatrists.

Failure to predict violence has nothing to do with how conservative we are, or with our clinical abilities. Consistently accurate prediction of any rare event is a mathematical impossibility under any set of remotely reasonable assumptions about the accuracy of the predictor. Ignorance of these mathematical facts almost certainly contributes to psychiatrists' belief that they can predict violence. To dispel the belief, we must explicate the statistical argument, although this has been done before (3).

Suppose that a psychiatrist is asked to predict whether every patient that he evaluates or treats will kill someone within one year or not. Or, suppose an investor is given a list of stocks and is asked to predict which ones will double in price within one year. Or, suppose a health inspector is asked to predict which restaurants he inspects will be responsible for salmonella-caused diarrhea in their customers within the next year.

In each of these three cases there is a body of knowledge and expertise that is relevant to the decision-making process. Let us assume further in each case that the person making the predic-

Table 1. Success of Prediction of Any Event When the Base Rate is 50 Percent and Accuracy is 95 Percent

	Actual Event		
	Positive	Negative	Total
Prediction			
Positive	475	25	500
Negative	25	475	500
Total	500	500	1,000

tions is an expert, and that he or she is able to predict with 95 percent accuracy; that is, that 19 of every 20 predictions will be correct. With these background facts known, let us consider the crucial variable: the base rate of occurrence of the event in question. First, let us suppose that the base rate is 50 percent. Under this assumption, one-half of the psychiatrist's patients will kill someone, one-half of the stocks will double, and one-half of the restaurants inspected will cause a salmonella outbreak. Let us assume, finally, that we have a sample of 1,000 cases for each example.

Table 1 illustrates how successful the predictions would be when the base rate is 50 percent and accuracy is 95 percent. The Table shows that 19 of 20 predictions are correct. Examining the positive predictions first, the psychiatrist would correctly predict, and presumably help prevent, 475 of 500 killings. The investor would successfully identify 475 of 500 stocks that would double and presumably he would become rich, and the restaurant inspector would prevent 475 outbreaks of salmonella. Twenty-five killings would occur; 25 good investments would be missed; and 25 outbreaks of salmonella diarrhea would occur. Examining the negative instances, we find identical results: 19 of 20 predictions are correct. Twenty-five patients would be incorrectly identified as potential killers, and presumably some preventive action would be taken; 25 stocks would be purchased and fail to double, and 25 restaurants would be unnecessarily asked to close down to take remedial action to prevent salmonella outbreaks.

Now, let us consider the same examples, but with a different base rate. Suppose that our accuracy remains the same, 95 percent,

Table 2. Success of Prediction of Any Event When the Base Rate is Two Percent and Accuracy is 95 Percent

	Actual Event		
	Positive	Negative	Total
Prediction			
Positive	19	49	68
Negative	1	931	932
Total	20	980	1,000

but that the event we are asked to predict is uncommon; the base rate is two percent rather than 50 percent. Under this assumption, 20 of the psychiatrist's patients would kill, 20 stocks would double, and 20 restaurants would be responsible for salmonella outbreaks. Table 2 presents the results under this set of assumptions. For the Table as a whole, 95 percent of predictions are correct, but there has been a major change for both positive predictions and negative predictions. In the case of positive predictions, only 19 of 68, or 28 percent, are correct. For every 68 people whom the psychiatrist thinks would kill, only 19 would have, and 49 would not have. Only 28 percent of the stocks selected would double, and only 28 percent of the restaurants closed as health hazards would have produced disease had they been permitted to remain open. In contrast, the accuracy of the negative predictions is greatly increased. Of 932 negative predictions, 931 are correct. We have incorrectly failed to institutionalize only one killer, have missed only one good stock, and have permitted only one salmonella outbreak. We have, however, interfered in the lives of many people who were not potential killers, bought many stocks that did not do as well as we expected, and closed many restaurants unnecessarily. Clearly, the social consequences of errors in prediction are a function of what we are trying to predict, but the proportion of correct predictions of positive and negative instances is entirely a function of base rates, once we have made an estimate of accuracy. Now, let us consider psychiatrists' predictions of potential violence as these relate to the *Tarasoff* duty.

In Chapter Two we reported eight *Tarasoff* cases involving patients in ambulatory treatment. These eight cases involved four killings: three by shooting, and one motor vehicle homicide; three non-fatal shootings, and one case of arson. There were 22,500 murders in this country in 1981, and 21,000 in 1982 (4). Assuming a population of approximately 171,000,000 adults, and assuming that each murder was committed by a different person, approximately one of every 8,000 Americans murdered someone else. Outside California (5), mental patients without a criminal record are no more likely to be violent than are other Americans (6). We will take as our base rate of murder one in 8,000.

The number of aggravated assaults (defined as attacks causing severe bodily injury, often with weapons) in this country was 644,000 in 1981 and 650,000 in 1982 (4). As a rough estimate, that is approximately four per thousand. A reasonable estimate of the likelihood of the type of violence from which failure to protect may lead to a suit is one in 500.

It is difficult to make an estimate of predictive accuracy based on anything except intuition. Years ago, when I worked for the federal government, we would be called upon to estimate unknown parameters, usually for important people. Sometimes we had some factual basis for an estimate, and sometimes not. On these latter occasions we used a procedure called SWAG. This stood for scientific wild ass guess. Absent any knowledge, we would "swag it." Swagging psychiatrists' predictive accuracy, I offer 95 percent, which I suspect is generous. The results of predicting under these assumptions are shown in Table 3. Table 3 assumes 10,000 cases in order to have whole numbers in the example.

Table 3 shows that the positive predictions are now correct in only 19 of 518 cases, or fewer than four times in 100. By contrast, the negative predictions are now essentially always correct. To prevent 19 episodes of major violence, the psychiatrist will attempt to protect the potential victim in over 500 cases.

This analysis helps to clarify why psychiatrists believe they can predict major violence. There is only one outcome that would convince psychiatrists they could not predict violence: the case in which the psychiatrist predicts no violence, and violence occurs. The Table shows that this occurs exactly one time in 10,000. The

Table 3. Success of Psychiatrists' Predictions of Major Violence by Their Patients When the Base Rate is 0.2 Percent and Accuracy is 95 Percent

	Actual Violence		
	Positive	Negative	Total
Predicted Violence			
Positive	19	499	518
Negative	1	9,481	9,482
Total	20	9,980	10,000

one case that would shake psychiatrists' belief in themselves occurs so rarely that most psychiatrists never experience it.

The Table also illustrates that it is not necessary to postulate a conservative predictive posture on the part of psychiatrists to explain the large number of false positives; that is, cases that are predicted to involve major violence when in fact none would have occurred. The large number of such cases is explained simply as a consequence of the low base rate of positive cases. Even when the psychiatrist's accuracy is 95 percent, five percent errors on the large number of negative cases must be a large number relative to 95 percent on the correctly predicted positive cases. In summary, the low base rate of major violence explains why psychiatrists are unable to predict violence with sufficient accuracy to be accurate in individual cases, and why psychiatrists believe that they can do so.

Notwithstanding all of the above, psychiatrists' intuition and society's faith may still be justified. Perhaps we can predict violence. The one unknown in our analysis is the correct estimate of psychiatrists' predictive accuracy. If 95 percent is correct, or even if the correct figure is 80 percent, then assuming that a psychiatric prediction permits some intervention of practical value, psychiatric prediction is of value in helping to prevent somewhere between 16 and 19 of every 20 people from being killed by their patients. This seems to be a highly desirable social goal.

Finally, we come to the end of this statistical analysis and logical argument. We now see why, even if psychiatrists can predict violence, the studies show that they cannot. The correct positive predictions are outweighed by the false positive predictions, so that in the individual case one has no way of knowing whether the individual would or would not have been violent. However, if we can predict violence as we believe, then we are preventing most major violence by our entire sample of patients; although it is impossible to determine whether in any given case we are preventing violence, or unnecessarily interfering in someone's life who would not have been violent in any case.

Whether we can predict violence accurately for samples of our patients is an empirical question that will not be answered for ethical reasons. In order to answer this question the research design would require that we predict violence, and then do nothing but sit back and observe whether it occurs. Given our belief that these predictions are accurate, such an experiment is morally untenable. We will have to search for approximate answers through other means, perhaps through laboratory experiments involving simulations or manipulation of related variables.

Society expects psychiatrists to predict potential major violence, I believe, because people have believed our historical claims that we can predict violence; and, also, because they believe that the social cost of these predictions in lives unnecessarily interfered with, is worth the gain in potential violence presumably prevented. Believing as I do in my own ability to predict violence and in that of many of my colleagues, I think that society's judgment is sound.

The implications of this analysis for clinical practice are substantial. The first conclusion is that none of us knows whether we can predict violence or not, although most of us believe we can. There is almost certainly a range of ability to predict violence among psychiatrists, and none of us can predict perfectly. Therefore, all of us must expect to be wrong sometimes if we make these predictions. Clearly, we will be wrong far more often in one way (needlessly interfering) than in the other (failing to act when we should).

The major consequence of this analysis is that the best protection against being accused of negligence at some point in one's career is to evaluate potential violence using a standard of care and a method of procedure that will be consistent with the highest professional standards and with all that we know about variables associated with violence.

This analysis makes clear that the clinician who relies on his clinical judgment, skill, or intuition to assess potential violence, but who fails to document how he or she has done this, or has failed to proceed in accordance with high standards of practice, puts himself or herself at risk of being found negligent should violence occur or should a patient claim that confidentiality has been inappropriately breached. It is grandiose to believe that one will always be right. One will often be wrong, and acceptance of that fact leads to professional humility: something I have understood and struggled to integrate in the course of writing this chapter.

There are a number of personal and social variables associated with violence (2). Being male, age 15–35, unemployed, and having a history of violence and alcohol or drug abuse, are all associated with violence. Situational variables that are associated with violence include having a violent environment, an unstable family, a peer group that is violent, available victims, and available weapons.

Clinical variables that are associated with violence include low intelligence, soft neurologic signs, paranoid suspiciousness, psychosis, anger and agitation, and the expressed wish to hurt or kill someone (7). If the clinician carefully assesses these variables and documents that assessment, and should the clinician's assessment of potential violence prove to be wrong, the likelihood of being found to have acted responsibly is increased, and the likelihood of being found negligent is correspondingly diminished. The careful assessment of potential violence is one aspect of the clinical response to *Tarasoff*, a subject which is dealt with more fully in Chapter Six.

References

1. Cocozza J, Steadman H: The failure of psychiatric predictions of dangerousness: clear and convincing evidence. Rutgers Law Review 29:1048–1101, 1976

2. Monahan J: The Clinical Prediction of Violent Behavior. Rockville, MD, National Institute of Mental Health, 1981

3. Rosen A: Detection of suicidal patients: an example of some limitations in the prediction of infrequent events. J Consult Psychol 18:397–403, 1954

4. FBI Uniform Crime Report, 1982. U.S. Dept. of Justice. Washington, D.C., 1983

5. Sosowsky M: Explaining the increased arrest rate among mental patients: a cautionary note. Am J Psychiatry 137:1602–1605, 1980

6. Rabkin JG: Criminal behavior of discharged mental patients: a critical appraisal of the research. Psychol Bull 86:1–27, 1979

7. Kroll J, Mackenzie TB: When psychiatrists are liable: risk management and violent patients. Hosp Community Psychiatry 34:29–37, 1983

6

Implications of *Tarasoff* for Clinical Practice

Paul S. Appelbaum, M.D.

6

Implications of *Tarasoff* for Clinical Practice

Previous chapters have reviewed the evolution of the legal duty to protect potential victims first enunciated in the *Tarasoff* decision, and have provided an overview of the effects of *Tarasoff* and its progeny on clinical practice. This chapter has a decidedly more practical emphasis. Few Court decisions have perplexed clinicians as thoroughly as have the opinions in *Tarasoff* and related cases. To be sure, there are many real difficulties with the *Tarasoff* doctrine as currently formulated, and the subsequent chapter will suggest a restructuring of the legal obligations incurred under the duty to protect. But the immediate need for clinicians is a practical guide for dealing with the law as it now exists. The following pages will attempt to ease the therapist's plight by offering a clinically-oriented model for fulfilling the *Tarasoff* duty. Strategies useful in the therapeutic setting will be outlined, and pitfalls noted.

Before proceeding with the analysis, a caveat is in order. *Tarasoff*-like cases have reached the appellate courts in only a

Parts of this chapter are drawn from an earlier discussion in Appelbaum PS: Tarasoff and the clinician: problems in fulfilling the duty to protect. *Am J Psychiatry* (in press, 1985).

minority of jurisdictions. Thus, most states have no law as to the applicability of the duty to protect. Even in states that have had court decisions on the subject, there has been a good deal of variation concerning some key aspects of the duty, as will be noted below. It is important to recognize, therefore, that this discussion is grounded in the assumption that, when faced with a *Tarasoff*-like case, given the momentum of the recent past, most jurisdictions will embrace some version of the duty to protect. Further, it is assumed that the duty in those cases will resemble in its essentials the model used in the mainstream of decisions to date. Before concluding that the model outlined here is appropriate for their jurisdiction, however, therapists are well advised to consult with local experts to ascertain any peculiarities in the law of their states.

A MODEL FOR UNDERSTANDING THE DUTY TO PROTECT

A significant part of the problem both Courts and clinicians have had in dealing with *Tarasoff*-like situations has arisen from the failure to recognize that the duty to protect patients' potential victims is, in reality, multifaceted, with three component parts. The duty requires the therapist to: 1) assess the patient's degree of dangerousness; 2) select a course of action to deal with the threat represented by the patient; and 3) implement that course of action appropriately. The components of the duty to protect will be considered in turn.

Assessment of Dangerousness

The first element of the duty to protect is the obligation to assess patients' potential dangerousness. Actually, this component of the duty itself is composed of two parts: gathering sufficient information with which to make a determination of dangerousness, and making the prediction.

Gathering information about potential dangerousness is, in

most cases, an integral part of the patient's routine evaluation. Therapists taking a history from a new patient will, as a matter of course, question the person about relationships with others, often leading to the revelation of material concerning outbursts of temper or physical altercations. A chronological recounting of the person's major life events will usually expose significant Court involvements or any substantial period of time spent in a penal institution. To the extent that a threatened loss of physical control is related to the patient's current difficulties, patients themselves will usually discuss these concerns spontaneously. Thus, in most cases, the initial *Tarasoff* obligation is fulfilled in the conduct of the routine assessment.

One additional step will complete the first stage of the duty to assess in almost all cases. Many clinicians have been taught to inquire directly about patients' past violent behavior while conducting a formal mental status examination (1). Given the current concern with the possibility of patient violence, it would be a wise precaution for all clinicians to adopt this practice. In addition, the information revealed will often be extremely relevant to the patient's evaluation, and should probably be obtained even in the absence of a legal obligation. Two simply worded questions accomplish this task. Patients can be asked: "Have you ever seriously injured another person?" and "Do you ever now think about harming someone else?" Therapists who routinely employ this approach will often confess their surprise at the information yielded by direct questioning, but not uncovered by the taking of a general history.

Most patients will lack histories of significant violence and current preoccupations with harming others. For them, the *Tarasoff* obligation, in its most reasonable interpretation, ends at this point. Other patients, however, will admit to violent acts or fantasies, or may during the course of treatment reveal desires to harm others. In these cases, the duty to gather appropriate information involves a more extensive assessment. The precise contours of what constitutes an adequate assessment are uncertain at present, given the controversy over therapists' abilities to predict dangerousness discussed in Chapter Three. Nonetheless, some general consensus exists in the literature on the subject as to what information is ordinarily relevant to the task.

Three areas of assessment are highlighted repeatedly. First, it is agreed that a small number of factors have been shown to be related statistically to the likelihood of future violence. These include: past history of violent behavior; age; sex; race; socioeconomic status; history of drug or alcohol use; intelligence and education; and residential and employment stability (2). Second, several authors have noted that one must assess the patient's psychological functioning insofar as it relates to conditions that are likely to decrease ability to control violent impulses (for example, command hallucinations), or to factors that are likely to increase internal controls (for example, obsessional defenses) (2, 3). Finally, the evaluating clinician should consider environmental circumstances that are likely to provoke or inhibit the expression of violent impulses, and in particular those that might interact with the psychological factors previously explored (4). Obviously, clinicians from different theoretical schools will focus on different indicators within each of the latter two areas. But standards of care are typically framed according to individual theoretical orientations; that should not pose a major problem here.

Admittedly, it is not possible to define with precision the extent of information-gathering that Courts may retrospectively determine to have been warranted in a particular situation. A Federal Court in California concluded that a recent violent act obligated assessing psychiatrists to attempt to obtain the patient's previous hospital records (which would have revealed an additional history of violence) even without the patient's consent (5). This seems an extreme position. The best protection for therapists from liability for a patient's future violence lies not in attempting to predict what irrational posture Courts may adopt in a particular case, but in gathering sufficient information to satisfy a standard of reasonable clinical care.

The most common mistake clinicians make during the information-gathering stage is gathering insufficient information on which to base a later determination of dangerousness. Usually this occurs because the therapist has a distorted understanding of the

Tarasoff obligation, assuming that the mere issuance of a threat by a patient or the commission of a threatening act necessitates action to protect future victims.

Case Example 1

A young paranoid schizophrenic woman called and harassed a local television personality from a telephone on an inpatient unit. Questioning of the patient revealed that she believed the man had slept with her mother and raped her sister. The resident in charge of her care sought consultation that he believed would confirm the need to call the object of the patient's delusions and warn him of potential danger. Instead, the resident was advised to assess more completely the patient's real threat to this man. It was pointed out that the patient's hospitalization on a locked ward allowed some leisure in gathering the necessary information. Inquiries directed to the patient's family revealed that the patient had been writing letters to and telephoning the broadcaster for five years, but had never made an overt threat or attempted to harm him. When questioned directly, the patient strongly denied that she had ever considered physical assault, although she admitted that she might continue her annoying telephone calls. The resident concluded that violence was very unlikely and no warning need be issued.

In fulfilling the duty to protect, the clinician is not compelled to act as a passive conduit for a patient's threats or mechanically to warn everyone in contact with a patient who once uttered a threat or committed a violent act. Rather, the therapist is charged with determining the likelihood of future violence and acting only when that likelihood is high. Many patients, particularly those with chronic psychotic illnesses, will offer threats against other persons who have been incorporated into their delusional systems, yet have no intention of ever acting to harm those persons. The obligation to assess encompasses the duty to gather sufficient information to separate those individuals who are likely to be harmless from those who represent a more substantial risk, before proceeding with the remaining elements of the *Tarasoff* duty.

Once appropriate information has been gathered, the duty to assess requires a determination of the patient's likely dangerousness. As discussed in Chapter Five, this is indeed a problematic task. Despite some consensus on what information is most relevant to determinations of future dangerousness, techniques for weighing that information to determine whether or not a patient presents a substantial risk of dangerousness are sorely lacking. In fact, the statistical argument presented in Chapter Five suggests that, given the low base rate of violence in our society, accurate predictions of future violence may never be attainable.

The Courts, however, have rejected these arguments repeatedly, choosing instead to hold therapists to a presumed professional standard of care in prediction. In the words of the *Tarasoff* Court, "the therapist need exercise that reasonable degree of skill, knowledge, and care ordinarily possessed and exercised by members of (that professional specialty) under similar circumstances" (6). Yet, in contrast to gathering information, for which standards do exist, there is no professional standard for predicting future violence. How is the clinician to respond to this seemingly illogical mandate?

The best approach to this situation is to make and document a *reasoned* decision about the patient's dangerousness. It matters less what particular basis is used for reaching the determination, than that there is an articulated rationale for the decision, preferably drawing on some recognized (even if empirically unvalidated) theory of causation of violence. Put more prosaically, the therapist can do no more than to think through the issue carefully and to do the best he or she can. The usual advice given in sticky clinical situations—to obtain the consultation of a supervisor or colleague —is useful here, as well. There is no better evidence that a clinician has attempted to adhere to the standard of care than written documentation that the views of colleagues (who in their collectivity establish the standard of care) were solicited.

It should be noted that what constitutes dangerousness is not always clear, either. Usually this term is taken to mean the likelihood of the patient assaulting another person. One recent case, however, found psychiatrists liable for permitting a patient with a chemical abuse history to continue driving a car, after the patient caused an accident in which other parties were injured (7).

Of course, there is no certainty in the process of determining dangerousness. A Court or jury in retrospect can always conclude that whatever process was used to arrive at the (by now obviously incorrect) determination that the patient was not likely to be violent was negligent. Again, however, clinicians cannot undertake their practice in fear of the rare, but disturbing, displays of unreasonableness by legal fact-finders. The opinion of the *Tarasoff* Court may provide some solace in this regard: "Within the broad range of reasonable practice and treatment in which professional opinion and judgment may differ, the therapist is free to exercise his or her own best judgment without liability; proof, aided by hindsight, that he or she judged wrongly is insufficient to establish negligence" (6).

Selecting a Course of Action

When a prediction of dangerousness has been made, the clinician must next select an approach that will be appropriately protective of potential victims. The *Tarasoff* decision imposed a duty to protect only identifiable victims; that is, those persons who are directly threatened by the patient or who "with a moment's reflection" the clinician can conclude are endangered (6). California Courts have explicitly rejected the position that therapists have an obligation to protect all persons who might be victims of the patient (8). Almost all jurisdictions that have adopted some form of the *Tarasoff* duty have concurred with this approach. There are Courts, however, that have extended the duty to the public at large (7, 9).

Although clinicians may not risk liability by failing to protect nonidentifiable victims (for example, when the patient threatens convincingly that he is going to leave the office, buy a gun, "and shoot the first person I see"), the next chapter will argue that there is little basis on moral grounds for distinguishing between the two situations. Thus, the approach outlined here is relevant to the protection of both identifiable and nonidentifiable victims.

As originally formulated in 1974, the *Tarasoff* decision established a "duty to warn," but explicitly required no other protective actions (10). Strong objections to the duty to warn from professional groups convinced the Court, when the case was redecided in 1976, that the duty should be framed more broadly: It concluded that the therapist "bears a duty to exercise reasonable care to protect the foreseeable victim" (6). Reasonable care need not involve warning, but in accordance with the intent of the decision, could encompass a wide range of other actions.

The psychiatric literature bears witness to the ingenuity of clinicians in responding to *Tarasoff*'s mandate to protect victims of patients' threatened violent acts (11-14). Options employed have included warning victims or alerting those who might exercise control over patients, such as the patients' relatives or the police. Patients have been hospitalized voluntarily and involuntarily. The emotions underlying patients' violent intent have been made an intensive focus of psychotherapeutic activity; medications have been used to help patients master their impulses, particularly when patients are psychotic. Therapists have expanded the traditional therapeutic dyad to include potential victims. Specialized forms of treatment, such as treatment for alcohol abuse, have been employed. Social service interventions have been useful in helping to stabilize or improve the patients' environmental circumstances. In short, the entire panoply of clinical interventions has been used by clinicians, in addition to the option of warning potential victims. A recent large-scale survey of therapists' practices, as well as smaller scale studies, have indicated that most therapists do, in fact, make use of this variety of approaches (13–15).

It would be impossible to offer a rigid system for matching appropriate responses to particular situations. Selecting a response requires as careful and skillful a consideration of individual needs and vulnerabilities as does any other intervention in treatment. Some rules of thumb, however, may be useful. In general, responses that are less disruptive to treatment should be selected over more disruptive alternatives. Thus, if potential victims can be protected reasonably well by alterations in the nature or focus of treatment (for example, the addition of medications or more frequent sessions designed to explore and defuse the patient's anger), such interventions should be preferred to responses that are directed outside of the therapeutic situation. If alterations in treatment are not likely to be sufficient, interventions that protect the patient's confidentiality (for example, offering to hospitalize the patient, or contacting a relative who is already aware of the patient's threats, so that the relative can supervise the patient or remove potential weapons from the environment) are preferable to actions that breach confidentiality (for example, calling the potential victim or the police). If confidentiality must be breached, in most circumstances this should be discussed first with the patient; clinical evidence suggests that this process helps to enlist the patient's observing ego in controlling his or her behavior, and minimizes later anger at perceived betrayal by the therapist. Obviously, when the therapist is afraid that open discussion would provoke an immediate attack on the victim or on the therapist, this most desirable interaction may have to be foregone. In fact, the most common difficulties clinicians encounter in the selection of a course of action relate to the failure to include the patient in the decision-making process (see Chapter Four). The benefits of enlisting the patient in the process are illustrated in the following case example.

Case Example 2

An 18-year-old man, in outpatient therapy for a borderline personality disorder and prominent antisocial traits, threatened to beat up his landlady after she refused to let her son associate with him. Assessing the threat, the therapist noted the patient's diffuse anger, based on an underlying sense of entitlement; his low level of impulse control; his susceptibility to psychotic regression; and his chronic use of alcohol and hallucinogens. Despite the absence of a past history of violent acts, the therapist was persuaded by the patient's repeated threats that the landlady was genuinely at risk.

At this point, the therapist shared his thoughts with the patient. He described the obligation he felt to avert the threatened assault, yet his reluctance to violate the confidentiality that had previously been an important part of the therapeutic relationship. Rather than making a decision on his own, the therapist invited the patient to comment on whether he would prefer hospitalization or some means of warning the landlady, the two most viable options at the time. The patient stated his desire to remain out of the hospital, but had no objection to the therapist calling the landlady to discuss the threat. This emphasized for the therapist the substantial manipulative component in the patient's original disclosure. A call was made to the landlady with the patient present, and the threat was revealed. The landlady responded that the patient had already voiced a similar threat to her directly, but that she was inclined to view it more as "blowing off steam" than as indicating that she was in serious jeopardy. In any event, she indicated, she knew how to take care of herself. After the call was made, the patient said that he would probably not have hurt her in any event. There were no subsequent ill-effects of the episode perceived in the therapy.

Here, bringing the patient into the decision-making process emphasized for him his responsibility for his own behavior. Patients who make threats in therapy, instead of acting on them directly, are often trying to transfer to the therapist the responsibility for controlling their impulses, and for the resulting consequences. Helping patients to recognize this process, and refusing to accept the delegated responsibility, is often a crucial part of treating character disordered patients.

Implementation of a Course of Action

It may seem axiomatic that whatever means are chosen to protect potential victims must be implemented appropriately. The things that can go wrong in the process, however, are illustrated by the following case example.

Case Example 3

A psychiatrist treating a woman who had, in therapy, threatened her supervisor at work, and misinterpreting the duty to protect, decided to warn the potential victim although he believed the threat was spurious. To effect the warning, he chose to write a letter to the personnel office of the organization for which the woman worked, revealing the threat she had made.

The psychiatrist's errors in this case were substantial enough to result in the only known verdict (in a suit for breach of confidentiality) against a clinician who has taken action to protect third parties (16). In addition to deciding to warn a victim despite his conclusion that she was not truly endangered, the psychiatrist chose the least appropriate means of implementing this course of action. His warning was sent by regular mail, a slow and uncertain means of communicating with a potential victim, and one that allows the recipient no opportunity to ask questions or provide feedback. Further, rather than sending the letter directly to the intended victim, the psychiatrist sent it through the personnel office, thus additionally slowing communication of the information and grossly breaching the patient's confidentiality. Warnings should ordinarily be communicated by telephone, although if the potential victim cannot be reached in that way, special delivery mail may be used. And, whenever possible, warnings should be given directly to the intended victim; a reliable third party can be employed as a go-between in those rare cases in which the victim is otherwise unreachable.

Implementation implies some degree of follow-up. If it is obvious to the clinician that the original course chosen to protect the potential victim is inadequate, further steps should be taken. This was precisely the situation faced by the therapists in *Tarasoff*. Having decided to commit their patient, they simply failed to take further measures to effect hospitalization when the patient was released by the university police. Obviously some limits to this principle must exist, otherwise therapists would be obligated to spend their days tracking down patients and former patients to assess the efficacy of protective interventions. In general, there should be only a limited obligation to follow up former patients who leave therapy after the intervention, or who were only seen in an evaluative context. That obligation should extend only to assuring oneself that the initial intervention was implemented effectively. Patients in ongoing treatment, however, should be followed more closely, with new strategies designed and implemented as necessary.

As will be discussed in the following chapter, some therapists have objected to the open-ended nature of the implementation component of the duty. They argue, largely correctly, that clinicians are not policemen and do not have the resources to track down patients or former patients to insure that protective measures continue to be effective. Yet, the *Tarasoff*-like cases to date have addressed only situations, like that in *Tarasoff* itself, in which the failure of the original plan was obvious to the therapists. Most reasonably interpreted, the duty to protect should require therapists to take further actions only when it is apparent in the normal course of following the patient that previous actions have been ineffective.

Particular problems arise when the care of the patients is transferred from one therapist or institution to another. Great care must be taken to insure that assessments and plans are clearly communicated between care-givers. When, for example, a patient is assessed as potentially violent and is hospitalized, the usual approach will be to reassess his or her dangerousness as discharge approaches to determine if further interventions are necessary. If the patient is transferred from one facility to another in the midst of hospitalization, as so often occurs, both the assessment of dangerousness and the need for re-evaluation should be communicated clearly to the new treatment team. Although written communications may be used for this purpose, direct telephone contact is preferable. Voice communication allows degrees of concern to be transmitted most effectively, and establishes a relationship between providers if recontact is later necessary. At least one *Tarasoff*-like case has already resulted in the imposition of liability, in part because of failure of communication between psychiatrists in the same facility (5).

CONCLUSION

The law has imposed substantial obligations on psychotherapists in recognizing their duty to protect their patients' potential victims. Although these obligations may be problematic in some ways—particularly when the Courts interpret them loosely in an effort to provide compensation, regardless of fault, to victims and their relatives (17)—in their most reasonable form they ought not to create unmanageable burdens for clinicians. Much of what the doctrine enunciated in *Tarasoff* requires would occur even in its absence, as a manifestation of good clinical care; this includes efforts to assess dangerousness, and in many cases the selection and implementation of effective responses. It is, after all, rarely in the interest of patients for them to be permitted to commit violent acts.

It would be wrong, however, to pretend that the duty to protect does not impose additional obligations, beyond those that were routine parts of clinical care in the past. Greater care must now be taken, and more extensive efforts made, in all three component areas of the duty: assessment, selection of a course of action, and implementation. There is no question, in addition, that the scope of therapists' potential liability has widened dramatically. Failures to undertake adequate assessment and treatment in the past were legal causes of action only if the patient suffered harm as a result and the patient or the patient's heirs sued. Under *Tarasoff*, clinicians' obligations extend to third parties, and more recently even those indirectly injured by the act of violence have been granted the right to compensation by the Courts (18).

Legal reforms are clearly necessary to prevent the more egregious abuses of the *Tarasoff* doctrine from continuing in the Courts. But, on the whole, clinicians have learned to live with *Tarasoff*, recognizing that good common sense, sound clinical practice, careful documentation, and a genuine concern for their patients, are almost always sufficient to fulfill their legal obligations.

References

1. Stevenson I, Sheppe WM: The psychiatric examination, in American Handbook of Psychiatry, 2nd ed, vol. 1. Edited by Arieti S. New York, Basic Books, 1974

2. Monahan J: The Clinical Prediction of Violent Behavior. Rockville, MD, National Institute of Mental Health, 1981

3. Gutheil TG, Appelbaum PS: Clinical Handbook of Psychiatry and the Law, New York, McGraw-Hill, 1982

4. Steadman JH: A situational approach to violence. Int J Law Psychiatry 5:171–186, 1982

5. *Jablonski v. U.S.*, 712 F.2d 391 (9th Cir. 1983)

6. *Tarasoff v. Regents of the University of California*, (Tarasoff II) 551 P.2d 334 (Cal. 1976)

7. *Petersen v. Washington*, 671 P.2d 230 (Wash. 1983)

8. *Thompson v. County of Alameda*, 614 P.2d 728 (Cal. 1980)

9. *Lipari v. Sears, Roebuck and Co.*, 497 F. Supp. 185 (D. Neb. 1980)

10. *Tarasoff v. Regents of the University of California*, (Tarasoff I) 529 P.2d 553 (Cal. 1974)

11. Roth LH, Meisel A: Dangerousness, confidentiality, and the "duty to warn." Am J Psychiatry 134:508–511, 1977

12. Wulsin LR, Bursztajn H, Gutheil TG: Unexpected clinical features of the *Tarasoff* decision: the therapeutic alliance and the duty to warn. Am J Psychiatry 140:601–603, 1983

13. Beck JC: When the patient threatens violence: an empirical study of clinical practice after *Tarasoff*. Bull Am Acad Psychiatry Law 10:189–201, 1982

14. Beck JC: Violent patients and the *Tarasoff* duty in private practice: does familiarity breed contempt? Presented at the Annual Meeting of the American Psychiatric Association, Los Angeles, May 11, 1984

15. Givelber D, Bowers W, Blitch C: *Tarasoff*, myth and reality: an empirical study. Wisconsin Law Review 1984: 443–497, 1984

16. *Hopewell v. Adibempe*, No. GD 78-28756, Civil Division, Court of Common Pleas of Allegheny County, Pennsylvania, June 1, 1981

17. Appelbaum PS: The expansion of liability for patients' violent acts. Hosp Community Psychiatry 35:13–14, 1984

18. *Hedlund v. Orange County*, 669 P.2d 41 (1983)

Rethinking the Duty to Protect

Paul S. Appelbaum, M.D.

7

Rethinking the Duty to Protect

In the last decade, psychiatrists have become greatly concerned about a growing number of Court decisions creating a legal obligation for them to protect potential victims of their patients' violent acts. The numerous critiques of these decisions, along with the varying approaches taken by Courts in different jurisdictions, suggest that although some agreement may exist on the moral underpinnings of the Court-imposed requirements, there is a good deal of controversy on the best means to achieve the desired goals. This chapter will review the problem created by the line of cases beginning with *Tarasoff*, which have established a therapist's "duty to protect," and will suggest an approach to this difficult area that balances the rights of society with the needs of patients and their therapists.

PROBLEMS CREATED BY THE DUTY-TO-PROTECT DECISIONS

The problematic consequences of the duty-to-protect decisions will be examined in four settings: prior to the initiation of therapy; during the usual course of therapy; when the therapist suspects the patient may intend to commit a violent act; and when a suit is brought alleging that the duty to protect has been breached.

Although empirical data relevant to the issues discussed in this section would be enormously useful in assessing the extent of the problems addressed, studies in this area have been rare, and many empirical efforts have had serious methodologic problems. Where empirical data exist, however, they will be noted in the discussion.

Problems Prior to the Initiation of Therapy

One of the primary concerns of psychotherapists has been that the decisions on the duty to protect will deter patients from seeking needed psychiatric care (1). This fear has arisen largely from a recognition that breaches of patient confidentiality—often in the form of warnings issued to potential victims—will be among the most frequent means chosen by clinicians to vindicate their responsibilities toward third parties. Since confidentiality has been assumed to be essential to persuading patients to enter psychotherapy (2), particularly when uncovering forms of therapy are employed (3), the fear that therapists may be compelled to reveal patients' angry feelings or hostile intentions toward others is thought likely to keep potential patients from the consulting room.

Empirical data relevant to this concern are sparse but suggestive. Although studies of the importance that patients and potential patients place on guarantees of confidentiality have shown mixed results, the more recent and methodologically sounder studies have indicated that patients place a high value indeed on the protection of their revelations (4–6). Nonetheless, the existing studies are not adequate to reveal whether patients faced with the options of no therapy or therapy only under the restrictions of the duty to protect would, in fact, decide to forego the benefits of psychotherapy. The reaction of potential patients may depend heavily on how much understanding they have of the scope and implications of the duty to protect. It may be argued that the majority of patients might not be deterred from entering therapy, but that a subgroup of persons struggling to maintain control over their violent impulses or misinterpreting the seriousness of their fantasies of violence would decline to participate in therapy when the risk of exposure exists. This would appear to be a reasonable assumption, even in the absence of supporting data.

A second probable effect of the duty to protect is to increase the likelihood that therapists, especially more experienced clinicians whose skills are in greater demand, will decline to treat potentially violent patients. The risk of liability and the need to transcend the usual realm of psychotherapeutic behavior by issuing warnings or taking other ill-defined steps to protect potential victims is likely to discourage therapists from becoming involved in the care of this problematic group of patients. Although it would be impossible for therapists to identify in advance all patients who raise such risks, patients with histories of violent acts or threats are likely to find themselves discriminated against.

Problems During the Usual Course of Therapy

Persuasive concerns have been voiced about the effects of the duty to protect during the course of psychotherapy. By heightening therapists' concerns with liability, the *Tarasoff*-like cases may well affect the manner in which therapy is conducted. Psychotherapists may, for example, place inappropriate emphasis on exploring patients' violent fantasies, when attention would be directed more appropriately to other areas of concern. One study of California therapists conducted soon after the initial *Tarasoff* decisions suggested that such a process might well be occurring (7). Conversely, the same study suggested that some therapists hesitate to investigate patients' angry feelings, which represent ubiquitous and often therapeutically important emotions, for fear that they might thereby uncover material that would necessitate some action on their part to protect potential victims. Either course of action, by distorting the usual therapeutic process, runs the risk of impairing the effectiveness of therapy.

Heightened therapist activity, of course, may well have effects that are not limited to considerations of potential violent behavior (7). The fear of liability and of having to meet a broad legal standard that encourages retrospective findings of negligence may interfere with the ability of psychotherapists to concentrate on patients' needs, particularly once the possibility of violence has been raised, and to deal with the extremely complex transference and countertransference issues that arise in the course of therapy.

Patients' behavior in therapy may also be altered by the duty to protect. Fearful of disclosure, patients may conceal information concerning their aggressive impulses, thus thwarting efforts to deal with them in therapy. The more uncomfortable the patient is with those impulses, and thus the more important it is that they be brought into the treatment process, the greater the possibility that they will be withheld. A number of psychiatric commentators have pointed to this phenomenon, along with the possibility that patients with violent impulses will be deterred from seeking therapy altogether, as constituting a paradoxical effect of the *Tarasoff* line of decisions: rather than insuring greater public safety, the duty to protect might increase the incidence of violent behavior by persons who avoided frank discussions of their impulses in therapy and therefore could not be treated satisfactorily (8).

When the Therapist Suspects the Patient May Commit a Violent Act

Clinicians have even greater concerns about the effects of the duty to protect at the point at which therapists' suspicions are raised about patients' potential for violence. The primary difficulty here involves severe limitations on the accuracy of clinicians' predictions of patients' future violent behavior. Although there was a time when psychiatrists felt sufficiently able to offer their services to the criminal justice system to assist in designing proper dispositions, that time has long past. For more than a decade, psychiatry and the other mental health disciplines have recognized that they have no particular expertise in the prediction of long-term violent behavior.

The studies that led to this conclusion are well summarized in recent publications (9) and thus do not require recapitulation here. Despite a variety of methodologic problems, every study performed in this area has demonstrated that mental health professionals have strikingly high false-positive to true-positive ratios (in the neighborhood of 4:1 to 3:1) when predicting long-term violence. Furthermore, given the rarity of violence in most populations, there is an impressive statistical argument that this tendency toward overprediction is unlikely to be overcome, even if highly accurate tests for violence are someday developed (10).

The situation with regard to prediction of violence over the short term is less certain. Studies are lacking in this area, and given significant ethical and legal problems with most conceivable study designs, it is not likely that they will be performed in the near future (11). Nevertheless, there is a feeling among many mental health professionals that they are able to predict with a fair degree of accuracy short-term (hours to days) as opposed to long-term (weeks to months) violence in psychiatric populations (12). This belief is based, in part, on the perception that accurate prediction of short-term violence involves an assessment of current mental states and their interaction with existing environmental circumstances, rather than the prediction of future mental functioning and environmental conditions. The former set of skills is probably much more within the capacity of mental health professionals, although even here, given low base rates of violence, the statistical argument still leads one to believe that accuracy will be limited.

Studies of psychotherapist behavior in the wake of *Tarasoff* have demonstrated another factor that is likely to limit predictive accuracy and favor overprediction (7; Chapter Three of this monograph). As a concomitant of heightened anxiety among therapists, respondents to these studies appear to have reduced their threshold for identifying patients as potentially violent. This is not surprising when one considers that the consequences of a failure to predict violent behavior that materializes (a false-negative prediction)—namely a dead or seriously injured victim and the possibility of a protracted lawsuit—are all the more salient for the therapist than those attending a prediction of violence that proves to be incorrect (a false-positive prediction). Unfortunately, this tendency to overpredict increases the likelihood that the adverse consequences described above will in fact occur, without a compensatory alteration in the level of protection afforded society.

Even in those cases in which accurate predictions are made, the therapist's ability effectively to prevent the violent act from occurring is limited. Warnings, the form of intervention most often associated with the duty to protect, are of dubious utility. Many potential victims are intimately involved with the patient, and are either already aware of the patient's violent tendencies, or are unlikely to remove themselves from the situation. Anecdotes from non-intimates who have been warned of a patient's violent intent indicate that it is extremely difficult to protect oneself from the possibility of assault (13, 14). One study of the effects of duty-to-protect cases found that responding clinicians reported no lower incidence of physical assault when warnings had been given than when they had not (See Chapter Three of this monograph).

There is reason to believe that actions taken within the context of ongoing therapy may be more effective than the issuance of warnings. Theoretical and anecdotal papers have indicated that involving the potential victim in therapy may be a useful approach (15, 16). Other alterations in the plan of therapy may also be of help (17). Voluntary or involuntary hospitalization, assuming the patient meets the commitment criteria in a given jurisdiction, represent additional alternatives. But the reality of overprediction, combined with the therapist's uncertainty as to which measures will be truly effective, mean that unnecessarily intrusive but potentially more secure alternatives (such as involuntary commitment) will frequently be chosen. Reports already exist of inappropriate hospitalization as a result of therapists' fears of liability (18); the resulting misuse of scarce resources and unnecessary loss of patient liberty are troubling but probably inevitable results of a broadly construed duty to protect.

Problems With Suits Alleging Breach of the Duty to Protect

Many of the difficulties plaguing application of the duty to protect in the clinical setting contribute to substantial problems in the adjudication of these cases. As noted earlier, the behavior of mental health professionals in predicting dangerousness is supposed to be measured by the usual standards of professional care. There may be elements of the duty to protect that lend themselves to such analysis, as will be described below, but efforts to apply professional standards to the prediction of future dangerousness are extremely problematic. Since the mental health professions openly acknowledge their incapacity to predict future dangerousness with any degree of accuracy, it is not clear that any standard at all exists for such behavior. Nor are the courts in a position to impose a standard of care, as they have in other areas of medical practice, such as informed consent (19), because they are equally at a loss to suggest how prediction might be accomplished.

The result of this absence of standards has been to encourage Courts to find defendants negligent based on the testimony of "experts" who declare, after the fact, that the patient's dangerousness should have been obvious to the therapists before the violence occurred. Clinicians, who are well aware of this phenomenon, are thereby forewarned that the safest course for them to follow is to predict dangerousness whenever the slightest indication is presented, compounding the problem of overprediction.

A related problem involves the failure of the Courts to define precisely what the duty to protect requires. To mandate that therapists take "whatever steps are reasonably necessary under the circumstances" may have intrinsic meaning for psychiatrists if the issue in question is the diagnosis of mental disorder; but this mandate provides no guidance to perplexed clinicians who have never been trained to protect persons from assault. This problem is exacerbated by the ruling in *Tarasoff* and later decisions that a lay standard of reasonableness, rather than a professional standard of behavior, should apply (20, 21). Since additional measures can *always* be taken, and there is no professional standard that can serve as a reference, therapists are left constantly in doubt as to whether their actions have been sufficient to encompass all that might be "reasonably necessary." Finders of fact at trial have equally little help from such a standard in determining the reasonableness of means chosen; there is a powerful tendency to conclude that the occurrence of violence must mean that all reasonably necessary steps were *not* taken. As currently formulated, therefore, the duty to protect constitutes a legal doctrine that is very difficult for the courts to administer.

A REASONABLE APPROACH TO THE DUTY TO PROTECT

It is my view that the objections to the duty to protect as currently formulated require a modification of the law that has evolved from the *Tarasoff* decision. With appropriate changes, I believe the duty to protect would be endorsed by most therapists, particularly if the argument is stripped of its polemical components. The following sections will present the moral and legal basis for my approach, and will elaborate my position in some detail.

An Overview of the Proposal

I begin by endorsing the moral obligation of clinicians to take appropriate protective actions when they believe that their patients pose a genuine risk to third parties. This position does not flow from any of the tort law maxims or precedents cited by the *Tarasoff* Court or the Courts that have adopted its reasoning. Rather, the recognition of this obligation stems from the belief that human beings in an organized society face a moral imperative to come to the assistance of their fellow human beings whose safety is endangered. Even if future Courts would unanimously reject the duty to protect, the moral obligation to which I refer would still exist.

There is evidence that this moral belief is widely shared by psychotherapists. Some of the harshest critics of the legal reasoning in the duty-to-protect cases have nevertheless endorsed some version of the duty on moral grounds (22). A survey of California psychotherapists not long after *Tarasoff* found that a substantial percentage had taken steps to warn or otherwise protect potential victims of their patients well before the law imposed such an obligation (7). A more recent and much larger nationwide survey of psychotherapists found broad acceptance of a moral duty to take protective actions, even among those who rejected the legal doctrine (Chapter Three of this monograph). In fact, the traditional rule of tort law that most persons owe no obligation to help their fellows in distress, to which *Tarasoff*-like cases represent uncommon exceptions, is probably anathema to most psychiatrists, other physicians, and other psychotherapists.

In theory, at least, a moral obligation of this sort need not lead to the imposition of a legal requirement. Courts are supposed to consider the consequences of alternative legal rules in formulating the duties to which they will hold defendants; they play a geniune policy-making role in this process. In practice, however, there is often no way to keep the moral obligation of a psychotherapist from being translated into legal standards. Faced with an allegation of negligence on the part of a mental health professional, the Courts determine its veracity by inquiring into the usual practices of that person's colleagues in similar situations. The process of translating commonly agreed upon standards of behavior into legally enforceable standards of care is often inexorable. In addition, society appears to have determined that therapists will be held accountable in Court for failures to protect third parties; guilt, adverse publicity, and the sanction of colleagues have been deemed inadequate responses, particularly insofar as they offer no compensation to the aggrieved victim. Thus, the nature of the legal rules that would enforce the moral and societal duty must be considered.

The position I am suggesting will be stated briefly here and then elaborated in the following sections of this chapter. In order to provide a clearly and reliably defined threshold for the invocation of psychiatrists' duties in this area, I urge that the duty to protect be invoked only when a patient threatens violence or commits a violent act that there is reason to believe may be repeated. The resulting duty should be fourfold: 1) to collect information revelant to an assessment of the patient's likely dangerousness, according to accepted professional standards; 2) to determine whether or not the patient is likely to be dangerous to others, according to procedures that do not show a reckless disregard for the information available; 3) to select a course of action; and 4) to implement that course of action, both according to accepted professional standards.

The Threshold Requirement: An Act or Threat of Violence

Many of the difficulties created by the duty to warn stem from the problems mental health professionals have in knowing when it should be invoked. A large number of patients have histories of past violence, some in the recent past; many others express violent fantasies in therapy sessions. Still more express feelings of anger, without clear ideas of acting on them. At present it is unclear which of these behaviors, if any, is sufficient to require the therapist to undertake the obligations associated with the duty to protect.

The Courts have had a deceptively simple answer for this question. Beginning with the *Tarasoff* decision itself, they have invoked the duty to protect "when the therapist determines, or pursuant to the standards of his profession should determine, that his patient presents a serious danger of violence to another . . . " (21). As we have seen, however, there are no accepted professional standards for the prediction of dangerousness; in fact, current knowledge provides no indication that reasonably accurate predictions are possible. Clinicians are therefore caught in a logical Catch-22: their duties to protect are only invoked when they know or should know that their patient will be violent, but the research literature suggests that they can never approach that state with any degree of confidence.

One might expect legal fact-finders to be equally perplexed as to when liability for failure to fulfill *Tarasoff*-like duties should be imposed on therapists. The Courts, however, have had an easy way out of this dilemma. Since they are operating with the benefit of hindsight, judges and juries face an all-too-often irresistible temptation to scrutinize records of treatment in search of some indication of potential dangerousness. For many patients, particularly those who later commit violent acts, such indications are easy to find. With support from an expert witness, who is aided by the same retrospective certainty, fact-finders can easily conclude that therapists should have known that the patient had the potential for violence.

In such circumstances, empirical evidence suggesting that therapists have been decreasing the level of suspicion at which they will take steps to protect third parties, and that they have altered their usual therapeutic practices to pursue even hints of potential violence, come as no surprise. The lack of a clear threshold of suspicion at which point the duty is invoked thus contributes to overprediction of dangerousness, needless breach of confidentiality and disruption of treatment, and an unfair standard of behavior by which therapists of violent patients are judged.

Society has faced a similar problem in another area of mental health law. For reasons of policy, the legislatures of most states have, since the late 1960s, altered their civil commitment statutes to restrict involuntary hospitalization to patients who are dangerous to themselves or to others (23). Like the *Tarasoff* Court, these legislatures have chosen this course in spite of powerful arguments that psychiatrists and other mental health professionals have great difficulties with the prediction of future violence. Unlike most of the duty-to-warn decisions, however, many legislatures have provided safeguards to limit, if not prevent, overprediction of dangerousness. These legislatures have restricted commitment to circumstances in which patients have engaged in an overt act of violence that is likely to be repeated (past violence being the single best predictor of future violence), or have made a convincing threat of violent action (24). Some states add that the act or threat must have been made in the recent past (25). By this means, patients are protected from the consequences of overprediction, and clinicians need not fear that every patient they fail to hospitalize will, if their clinical judgment was incorrect, provoke charges of malpractice.

I believe, for similar reasons, that an analogous threshold should exist in duty-to-warn cases. Therapists should not be held liable for failure to fulfill the elements of the duty to warn outlined below, unless patients have engaged in violent behavior or made threats of violence in the recent past. I am gratified and encouraged that two Courts have already come to this conclusion independently (26, 27). This threshold requirement was also tacitly embodied in many of the pre-*Tarasoff* release-and-escape cases, in which liability, even for negligent release, was rarely imposed in the absence of foreseeable behavior, as demonstrated by an overt act or threat of violence.

It should be noted that an even more restrictive threshold has been suggested. Responding to the "special relationship" analysis in *Tarasoff*, built in part on psychotherapists' ability to control patients through the involuntary commitment process, some commentators have suggested that only patients who are in fact committable—that is, whose behavior can truly be controlled—should trigger the duty to protect (22). Although the logic is appealing, I reject this approach as unduly restrictive. State commitment statutes vary widely. Those with broader commitment criteria will not materially limit the scope of the duty to protect. Those with more stringent criteria may limit it unduly. Some states, for example, exclude threats as a basis for commitment, requiring action to accompany them (25). That seems an unreasonable narrowing of the duty to protect. In addition, since commitment criteria are likely to continue to change in the future, if we conclude that the duty to protect has an independent moral basis, it seems unwise to link it to criteria for commitment that cannot be specified at this time.

The question of whether the threshold requires that an act or threat be directed against an identifiable victim must also be addressed. The decisions in *Tarasoff* and most of its progeny have limited the duty to protect to readily identifiable victims of the patient. Convincing arguments have been presented, however, concerning the limitations of this approach (28). It makes little sense to differentiate, if a moral duty is at stake, a case in which the patient clearly identifies the victim, from a case in which a convincing threat of violence is made but the name of the victim is omitted. Both named and unnamed victims are human beings whose welfare ought to be a concern of the patient's therapist. Courts that have attempted to make this distinction, as some have (29), have strained the bounds of logic to do so. Other Courts have simply interpreted identifiability with such latitude as to create a parody of the rule (30). Although it is true that discarding the identifiable victim criterion broadens the scope of potential liability for the psychotherapist, logic and moral considerations seem to require this step.

Finally, I am not suggesting that psychiatrists be precluded from taking protective actions if convinced of their patients' dangerousness, unless the threshold of an act or threat has been crossed. There may be circumstances in which, in the absence of either an act or threat, a therapist is persuaded of a patient's lethality. That a therapist would feel compelled to act in such a circumstance is understandable and commendable. But given the particular uncertainty of predictions in such situations, the therapist should not be required to take action for fear of liability.

The Duty to Protect—Information Gathering

Most of the extensive literature on the duty to protect has failed to recognize that the duty is composed in reality of four component parts. This analysis problem has contributed to the difficulty commentators have had in agreeing on standards by which therapists' behavior should be judged. For some components of the duty, it is entirely reasonable to assess clinicians' actions according to professional standards of care, while for others it is not.

The first component of the duty to protect involves gathering information relevant to the determination of dangerousness. This obligation goes beyond the routine questions most psychiatrists have been trained to ask about patients' past acts of violence, or current homicidal preoccupations. Once the threshold for the duty to protect has been triggered by a violent act or the threat of one, the therapist should be required to gather appropriate information for the evaluation of dangerousness, according to accepted standards of professional behavior. It may seem paradoxical that standards for information gathering can exist in the absence of agreement on whether future dangerousness is currently predictable. In fact, the paradox is illusory: consensus can be achieved as to which information allows the best possible predictions of dangerousness to be made, even as we acknowledge that those predictions are often highly inaccurate. The preceding chapter provides an indication of the nature of the current consensus on which information is relevant to the determination.

Clinicians who fail to live up to a reasonable professional standard with regard to data gathering for the assessment of dangerousness may be found to have behaved negligently. Ultimate liability, of course, will still be dependent on proof of injury and proximate cause. It is of interest that some of the *Tarasoff*-like cases have faulted clinicians not for failing to predict dangerousness, but for failing to accumulate appropriate data with which to assess the likelihood of violence (31).

The Duty to Protect—Prediction of Dangerousness

The most frequently discussed component of the duty to protect is the obligation to determine whether or not the patient is genuinely dangerous. Currently insuperable difficulties with predictions in this area have been addressed at length above. Some commentators have argued on this basis that the duty to protect as a whole ought to be abandoned, since it is meaningless to ask therapists to control those whom they cannot identify. Unfortunately, the matter is not that simple.

Justice Mosk of the California Supreme Court recognized this problem in his concurrence and dissent in the 1976 *Tarasoff* decision. He argued that, in the absence of meaningful professional standards for the prediction of dangerousness, it was poor policy to hold therapists liable for failing to make predictions in accordance with those standards. Rather, Justice Mosk and others (22) would hold therapists liable only when the therapists first conclude, on whatever basis, that their patients are likely to be dangerous to others, and then fail to take appropriate measures to protect the victims.

Although this approach has much to commend it, I am concerned with its limitations. Such a rule fits well with the facts in *Tarasoff*, but it will be rare that clear-cut documentary evidence exists that a therapist has determined a patient to be dangerous and then failed to act. The acceptance of Mosk's approach might even encourage therapists to avoid coming to conclusions about or documenting patients' potential dangerousness, in the hope that these measures would provide protection against successful suits; either defensive technique would represent poor clinical practice.

More significantly, there will always be cases in which the evidence of a patient's potential for violence seems so clear, even given current uncertainties, that a clinician's decision to ignore it is nothing less than outrageous. Such might be the case if a psychotic patient who had, on instructions from hallucinated voices, assaulted several people just prior to his evaluation, were to be sent home without medications or plans for treatment, because the clinician did not believe that further violence was likely. That the clinician in this case might be immune from liability under Mosk's approach weighs heavily against it.

Instead of the Mosk rule, I support a standard that would recognize the absence of professional guidelines for prediction, yet allow remedies to be obtained in cases of outrageous neglect of professional and common sense. I would favor limiting the imposition of liability for failure to fulfill this element of the duty to protect only if the clinician acted in *reckless disregard* of the available evidence. This standard has several advantages. First, by moving away from the nebulous "professional standard" approach for this component of the duty, it allows additional leeway to clinicians in the uncertain matter of prediction of dangerousness. The pressure to practice "defensive psychiatry," involving the overprediction of dangerousness and the taking of inappropriate actions to protect victims, will thereby be mitigated. Second, courtroom determinations of a breach of this component of the duty will no longer rest on expert testimony about nonexistent standards, shaped to the peculiar facts of the case.

Nor will the Courts have to pretend that clear-cut standards exist; they will thus rid themselves of the taint of hypocrisy when, in order to provide reimbursement to victims, they declare that those standards have not been met. On the other hand, the reckless disregard standard will offer protection to the public from unquestionably negligent behavior of clinicians, while putting the latter on warning that good-faith efforts must be made when dealing with potentially dangerous patients. This probably represents the best compromise in this area, whereby clinicians who have been asked to assume the additional, extra-therapeutic task of safeguarding society are given a substantial amount of flexibility in carrying out the most difficult aspect of that role.

Duty to Protect—Selecting a Course of Action

When a clinician determines that a patient is likely to be violent toward others, the duty to protect, as embraced here, requires the clinician to take reasonable steps to safeguard potential victims. The reasonableness of the course of action selected should be judged by a professional standard of care; that is, what other clinicians similarly situated would have chosen to do in these circumstances.

As noted above, it has been argued that thus formulated the duty to protect is too ill-defined to allow clinicians to know when they have or have not satisfied its requirements (22). Alternatives have been discussed, including requiring only that therapists issue warnings, the original (1974) *Tarasoff* position, or requiring only that they hospitalize the patient, if that option is available. Although a more broadly formulated duty places clinicians at increased risk—since no single action can be said in advance definitively to fulfill the duty—I favor the broader approach as less disruptive to patients' clinical care. Limiting therapists' choices to warning potential victims will encourage them to breach confidentiality when more clinically oriented approaches, including modifications in the treatment plan, would achieve a higher level of protection, and simultaneously meet patients' needs. Limiting therapists' choices to committing patients will encourage over-commitment, with its accompanying misuse of valuable mental health resources, while not addressing the protection of potential victims of non-committable patients.

The implicit goal of these narrower approaches—to place acceptable limits on therapists' potential liability—can in fact be accomplished within a "reasonable care" model. As long as therapists are held to a genuine professional standard of care—in contrast to *Tarasoff*'s lay standard—as they are in all other areas of clinical practice, they should be able to select any reasonable option or combination of options with the assurance that liability will not ensue. Sufficient information is becoming available from empirical studies and anecdotal reports to indicate what the scope of reasonable professional practice might be (See Chapter Three of this monograph). Clinicians will undoubtedly be relieved to know that these data suggest that the majority of their colleagues would choose, whenever possible, a clinically oriented intervention designed to decrease patients' potential dangerousness. I support this approach and would encourage clinicians to reserve warnings, with their inherent breach of patient-therapist confidentiality, for situations in which clinically oriented options are insufficiently protective of potential victims.

Duty to Protect—Implementation

The final component of the duty to protect requires therapists to implement appropriately the course of action they have chosen. Indeed, the *Tarasoff* case itself focused on this component of the duty. Poddar's therapists determined that he represented a danger to Tatiana Tarasoff and decided to seek his involuntary commitment. They requested that the police detain him, but when the police released Poddar, they did not pursue further actions to protect Tatiana Tarasoff. No questions have been raised about the propriety of the therapists' behavior in relation to assessment, prediction, or selection of a course of action. It was the therapists' alleged failure to implement their decision effectively that brought *Tarasoff* to court.

Of course, the *Tarasoff* case also demonstrates the difficulties that can arise in determining whether clinicians have taken reasonable steps to implement their decisions. Some may argue that asking the campus police to detain Poddar was all one could expect of the therapists; subsequent events should be attributed to the police's inexplicable decision to release him (22). (Consistent with other Court rulings, the *Tarasoff* Court ultimately granted the police immunity for their actions on policy grounds.) Again, however, the issue can best be resolved by utilizing a professional standard of care. Therapists should be required to use as much persistence in implementation as would a reasonable colleague in a similar situation.

Some of the earlier release-and-escape cases offer examples of the kinds of problems that are likely to arise at the implementation stage. Clinicians who agree to notify the Courts or potential victims when a patient is released and fail to do so may be at risk for charges of negligence (32). The failure to transmit relevant information to subsequent care-givers, who may be unaware of a patient's dangerousness or of the plans agreed on to manage it, may also create problems for therapists in this area (33).

It will be important, however, for Courts to recognize, in the words of some of the release-and-escape decisions, that therapists are not "guarantors" of the public's safety. The mere fact that a plan of action proved to be ineffective does not imply that there was negligence involved in its selection or implementation. Availability of resources, including alternative treatment facilities, support staff, time, and money, should also be taken into account in determining what constitutes reasonable behavior. A psychiatrist in an understaffed facility, responsible for the welfare of dozens of patients, cannot reasonably be expected to devote large amounts of time over a substantial period to follow up a single patient. Taking such limitations into account may sometimes frustrate the desire of the Courts to provide compensation to victims, but represents a just application of long standing and well-accepted principles of negligence.

CONCLUSION

Public policy concerning protection of potential victims of patients' violent acts has been difficult to formulate because of the varying interests that must be accommodated. The evidence suggests that mental health professionals have, for some time, been willing to accept responsibility for the protection of the public, as long as that obligation neither unduly interferes with the treatment of their patients, nor leaves clinicians at unreasonable risk of liability. I believe that the approach outlined above represents a reasonable compromise of these interests. Therapists will be encouraged to protect potential victims of their patients, but only when a recent act or threat of violence has occurred. Their actions will be judged by a professional standard of care, except for the prediction of dangerousness, an area in which no meaningful professional standards exist. These modifications of the duty to protect will limit disruption of psychotherapy and breach of patients' confidentiality, while providing protection to the public in those cases in which it is most likely to be needed.

References

1. Brief for Amici Curiae, American Psychiatric Association, et al., *Tarasoff v. Regents of the University of California*, 551 P.2d 334 (Cal. 1976)

2. Dubey J: Confidentiality as a requirement of the therapist: technical necessities for absolute privilege in psychotherapy. Am J Psychiatry 131:1093–1096, 1974

3. Hollender MH: Privileged communication and confidentiality. Diseases of the Nervous System 26:169–175, 1965

4. Lindenthal JJ, Thomas CS: Psychiatrists, the public and confidentiality. J Nerv Ment Dis 170:319–323, 1982

5. Schmid D, Appelbaum PS, Roth LH, et al: Confidentiality in psychiatry: a study of the patient's view. Hosp Community Psychiatry 34:353–355, 1983

6. Appelbaum PS, Kapen G, Walters B, et al: Confidentiality: an empirical test of the utilitarian perspective. Bull Am Acad Psychiatry Law 12:109–116, 1984

7. Wise TP: Where the public peril begins: a survey of psychotherapists to determine the effects of *Tarasoff*. Stanford Law Review 135:165–190, 1978

8. Stone AA: The *Tarasoff* decisions: suing psychotherapists to safeguard society. Harvard Law Review 90:358–378, 1976

9. Monahan J: The Clinical Prediction of Violent Behavior. Rockville, MD, National Institute of Mental Health, 1981

10. Livermore J, Malmquist C, Meehl P: On the justifications for civil commitment. University of Pennslyvania Law Review 117:75–96, 1968

11. Monahan J: Prediction research and the emergency commitment of dangerous mentally ill persons: a reconsideration. Am J Psychiatry 135:198–201, 1978

12. Monahan J: The prediction of violent behavior: toward a second generation of theory and policy. Am J Psychiatry 141:10–15, 1984

13. Halleck SL: Law in the Practice of Psychiatry. New York, Plenum Medical Book Co., 1980

14. Beck JC: Violent patients and the *Tarasoff* duty in private practice: does familiarity breed contempt? Presented at the Annual Meeting of the American Psychiatric Association, Los Angeles, May 11, 1984

15. Wexler DB: Patients, therapists, and third parties: the victimological virtues of *Tarasoff*. Int J Law Psychiatry 2:1–28, 1979

16. Wulsin LR, Bursztajn H, Gutheil TG: Unexpected clinical features of the *Tarasoff* decision: the therapeutic alliance and the "duty to warn." Am J Psychiatry 140:601–603, 1983

17. Roth LH, Meisel A: Dangerousness, confidentiality, and the duty to warn. Am J Psychiatry 134:508–511, 1977

18. Appelbaum PS: Hospitalization of the dangerous patient: legal pressures and clinical responses. Bull Am Acad Psychiatry Law (in press)

19. *Canterbury v. Spence*, 462 F.2d 772 (D.C. Cir. 1972)

20. *Tarasoff v. Regents of the University of California*, (Tarasoff II) 511 P.2d 334 (Cal. 1976)

21. *Petersen v. Washington*, 671 P.2d 230 (Wash. 1983)

22. Stone AA: Law, Psychiatry, and Morality. Washington, D.C., American Psychiatric Press, 1984

23. Appelbaum PS: Civil commitment, in Psychiatry, Epidemiology, Legal, and Social Psychiatry, vol. 5. Edited by Klerman G. Philadephia, J. B. Lippincott; New York, Basic Books (in press)

24. Dix GE: Major current issues concerning civil commitment criteria. Law and Contemporary Problems 45:137–159, 1982

25. *Pennsylvania Statutes Annotated*, Title 50, Section 7100 (1978)

26. *Brady v. Hopper*, 570 F. Supp. 1333 (D. Colo. 1983)

27. *Hasenei v. U.S.*, 541 F. Supp. 999 (D. Md. 1982)

28. Mills MJ: The so-called duty to warn: the psychotherapeutic duty to protect third parties from patients' violent acts. Behavioral Sciences and the Law (in press)

29. *Thompson v. County of Alameda*, 614 P.2d 728 (Cal. 1980)

30. *Davis v. Lhim*, 335 N.W.2d 481 (Mich. Ct. App. 1983)

31. *Jablonski v. U.S.*, 712 F.2d 391 (9th Cir. 1983)

32. *Semler v. Psychiatric Institute of Washington*, 538 F.2d 121 (4th Cir. 1976)

33. *Underwood v. U.S.*, 356 F.2d 92 (5th Cir. 1966)

8

Overview and Conclusions

James C. Beck, M.D., Ph.D.

8

Overview and Conclusions

WHAT IS THE *TARASOFF* DUTY, AND WHEN DOES IT APPLY?

Psychiatrists and other clinicians have always owed duties to patients. These are described in formal statements of professional ethics (1), and in case and statutory law. The *Tarasoff* decision (2) of the California Supreme Court enunciated a new duty for psychotherapists—a duty to protect possible victims of potentially violent patients. The *Tarasoff* decision failed to specify how the therapist should act, but left the choice to professional judgment. This decision superceded an earlier decision (3), which held that psychotherapists have a duty to warn the victim. Many clinicians continue to believe that warning is the only action that satisfies the legal duty, despite the Court's withdrawal from this position.

The California Legislature recently passed a bill that would have limited *Tarasoff* liability to situations in which the patient communicated a threat to the therapist, and the therapist failed to warn the victim. However, the Governor of California vetoed the bill. In his veto message he erroneously described the current law as requiring a warning (4). Once introduced, the idea of warning appears to hold a powerful grip.

To know when a Court is likely to hold that a *Tarasoff* duty applies, it is helpful to look at the decisions that have been published. California Courts have decided these cases rather differently from Courts in other jurisdictions. Cases involving outpatients have been decided differently from those involving discharged inpatients. In examining these four classes of cases, certain regularities emerge.

California Courts have decided two outpatient cases (5,6) and one inpatient release case (7). In both outpatient cases, the Court held that there was a foreseeable victim, and found the defendant negligent. In the inpatient case, the Court found that the victim was not foreseeable because he was not identified—in spite of the fact that the killer, a delinquent released from a county detention facility, had threatened to kill a child in the neighborhood, and then did so within 24 hours. Absent a foreseeable victim, the Court found for the defendant.

Outside California, no Court has applied the *Tarasoff* duty to an outpatient case, *and* found liability on the facts. There have been six outpatient cases outside California. In *McIntosh* (8), the Court held that *Tarasoff* applied, but found for the defendant. In *Peck* (9), the Court held that *Tarasoff* was not the law in its jurisdiction. In *Shaw* (10), the Court found that, absent a threat to an identified victim, *Tarasoff* was irrelevant. In *Brady* (11), the Court found that *Tarasoff* did not apply because there was no foreseeable victim. The final two outpatient cases involved suit, not for breach of *Tarasoff*, but for breach of confidentiality (12,13). In *Hopewell*, the Court said that *Tarasoff* was not the law, and found the defendant negligent (12). In *MacDonald*, the Court held that *Tarasoff* was the law (13), but the facts were never litigated. On this record, a psychotherapist outside California is more likely to be found negligent for breach of confidentiality (one case in 10 years), than for breach of *Tarasoff* (no cases in 10 years).

Outside California, there have been eight inpatient release cases. In three cases, the Court held that there was a *Tarasoff* duty (14-16), and in two of these the Court found the psychiatrist negligent (14,15). In *Davis* (14), the Court held that the victim was foreseeable, solely on the fact that the patient had threatened her three years earlier. In *Petersen* (15), although the Court said the psychiatrist had a duty to protect, there was no named victim, and the Court said the psychiatrist should have petitioned for commitment of his patient rather than release him. Thus, although the Court said this was a *Tarasoff* duty, as a matter of fact it was indistinguishable from the traditional fact situation of inpatient release cases, and the Court's remedy was the traditional one: hospitalize. The third inpatient case (16) involved a threat to one person, and has not yet been decided on the merits.

In five inpatient release cases outside California, the Courts held that either *Tarasoff* was not the law, or that the facts did not meet a *Tarasoff* standard. In all five cases there was no threat to a named individual, and in all five cases the Courts held that, absent a foreseeable victim, there was no negligence (17–21).

The foregoing analysis of recent case law clarifies instances in which a court is likely to invoke the *Tarasoff* duty. If the psychotherapist is treating an ambulatory patient, the *Tarasoff* duty begins to operate only after there is evidence, either from threats or acts, that the patient is dangerous to a specific, identifiable person. The danger involved must be substantial: serious bodily harm or death. If a careful clinical assessment fails to reveal a history of violent threats or actions against a specific identifiable person, a Court is unlikely to hold a psychiatrist or other psychotherapist to have violated his or her duty, should violence occur. The Courts appear to invoke *Tarasoff* in outpatient cases according to the standard suggested by Appelbaum in Chapter Seven.

The preceding analysis suggests that, in many inpatient release cases, the *Tarasoff* rule adds little or no additional burden on the psychiatrist or other mental health professional beyond that imposed by the traditional requirement that he or she practice according to usual professional standards. Logically, this is correct. If a dangerous person is released, and there is negligence, the negligence is not in failing to act appropriately after release, but rather in failing to appreciate the dangerousness before release. If the psychiatrist appreciated the dangerousness, and discharged the patient, clearly he or she would be liable for knowingly discharging a dangerous patient. The duty to protect would have been served by continued hospitalization. If the psychiatrist failed to appreciate the dangerousness, the success or failure of a suit would turn on whether the psychiatrist's evaluation met the usual standard of care.

One type of inpatient for whom the *Tarasoff* duty may be relevant is the person who is both schizophrenic and antisocial, and who has seriously threatened or assaulted an individual. If the schizophrenia is successfully treated and the patient petitions for release, he or she is likely to be released under current law in most jurisdictions. If the psychiatrist considers the patient still dangerous because of his antisocial personality, he or she should seriously consider warning any identified victim.

Another possible scenario in which a *Tarasoff* duty might apply to an inpatient occurs when the psychiatrist assesses the patient as dangerous, and petitions for commitment, but the Court then denies the petition—a fact situation analogous to that of Poddar's therapist. If the psychiatrist is in such a situation, he or she should make certain to introduce his or her concerns about potential violence on the record. The psychiatrist would be well advised to consider what additional steps to take.

To begin with, the psychiatrist should have a thoughtful discussion with the patient about his or her concerns and the patient's intentions, make a careful assessment of the patient's mental status, and consult with a trusted colleague or supervisor. Only then should the psychiatrist decide on a course of action. In the best case, the psychiatrist and patient will reach agreement on how to proceed. Perhaps they will agree to bring in the proposed victim for a three person discussion, or the therapist might telephone the victim with the patient present. In the rare case in which it is impossible to reach agreement with the patient, the therapist should acknowledge the disagreement, and apprise the patient of what he or she intends to do. In any such case, the therapist should write a careful, detailed note documenting his or her assessment, conclusions, and proposed course of action.

Psychiatrists and other psychotherapists owe a duty to safeguard the patient's confidentiality, as well as a duty to protect third parties. Ironically, the only successful suit involving the *Tarasoff* duty in an outpatient case was one in which the Court held that *Tarasoff* did not apply because of state statutes protecting confidentiality. The psychiatrist was held liable for breach of confidentiality (12). The psychiatrist appears to have been motivated, in part, by a desire to avoid the legal consequences of failing to warn. The resulting suit speaks to the importance of psychiatrists' making their judgments of whether *Tarasoff* applies on clinical, rather than on legal, grounds. In addition, every psychiatrist should know the law on confidentiality in his or her jurisdiction. Unlike the *Tarasoff* duty that only rarely arises, the duty to maintain confidentiality is constantly present in clinical practice. Breach of confidentiality occurs often in the practice of psychiatry, and the psychiatrist should know the relevant law.

The preceding analysis encompasses every case except *Lipari* (22), which is exceptional on several grounds. First, it is the only case involving a day patient rather than an outpatient or inpatient, so that the degree of control exercised by the therapist is intermediate between what is exercised in outpatient and inpatient cases. In outpatient cases, the courts have said that the therapist's control over the patient is not sufficient to establish a duty to protect, absent a foreseeable victim. In inpatient cases, the Courts have found that there is a duty to control with or without a foreseeable victim. Furthermore, although the patient was ambulatory, *Lipari* was more like inpatient release cases than typical outpatient cases, in that the patient had dropped out of treatment at the time of the crime. The holding, that the defendant owed a duty in the absence of an identified victim, is also unusual.

IMPACT OF *TARASOFF* ON PSYCHOTHERAPISTS

The relatively small number of published cases may underestimate the burden psychiatrists experience resulting from the *Tarasoff* duty. There may be other cases that are unpublished because they have been decided in lower courts, or because they were settled before coming to trial. The fact that the American Psychiatric Association (APA) legal consultation service receives more questions about *Tarasoff* cases than any other subject, certainly suggests that this is an ongoing source of concern to a greater extent than the number of psychiatrists actually found negligent would imply.

The small number of published cases and the large number of informal inquiries by psychiatrists to the APA, taken together, suggest that the *Tarasoff* decision has had a prophylactic effect. That is, psychiatrists are more attuned to possible dangerousness, and they act to prevent it. They are meeting their duty to third parties, and the result is relatively many consultations and relatively few successful suits.

Wise (23) found that psychiatrists' threshold for predicting dangerousness in California appeared to be dropping, and that the average California privately practicing psychiatrist saw 240 patients per year, 14 (or 5.8 percent) of whom were described as dangerous. Either there is much more murder and mayhem among Californians than they are letting on, or these psychiatrists have begun to regard as dangerous behavior that would not trigger a *Tarasoff* duty if it occurred. Givelber and his colleagues reported, in Chapter Three, that 45 percent of psychiatrists who had warned felt that they had compromised their professional judgment at some time in their careers, in contrast to just over 30 percent of those who had not warned anyone. It is a fair inference that in many instances psychiatrists are warning in spite of their best clinical judgment, not because of it.

These facts, taken together, suggest that psychiatrists are practicing defensively, and at times in opposition to their own best judgment. The recent legal cases suggest that the Courts are grappling responsibly with difficult clinical issues. For the most part, the Courts understand the issues and the profession. They do not have an idealized picture of psychiatrists, and they do not hold us to unrealistic, idealized standards. Almost always, outside California, they hold us to standards that seem reasonable. This analysis implies that good clinical judgment is the best defense against being sued. Trying to protect oneself by acting against one's better judgment will be counterproductive, since we must avoid the *Scylla* of breaching confidentiality on one side, and the *Charybdis* of failing to protect the victim on the other. As the analysis in Chapter Five makes clear, there is reason to believe that we can identify most potentially violent patients. If we rely on our clinical judgment and use good sense, we will serve our patients and society well, and protect ourselves in the bargain.

The survey data presented in Chapter Three suggest clearly that most therapists now regard the *Tarasoff* duty as an ethical responsibility as well as a legal duty. Furthermore, the *Tarasoff* duty has led very few psychiatrists to avoid dangerous patients.

CLINICAL IMPLICATIONS OF THE *TARASOFF* DUTY

The cases in Chapter Four illustrate one basic point. When the clinician integrates the *Tarasoff* duty into the clinical work, the effect on the therapy is either positive or neutral. The cases in which the therapist warns in a legalistic way, or warns without first discussing the warning with the patient, are cases in which the warning has a bad effect on the therapy, and in which there may be an associated poor outcome.

If a therapist believes, after careful assessment, that a particular patient represents a real and substantial threat of harm to another, then the therapist has an obligation to the patient as well as to the victim to prevent violence. Patients' proposed violent actions are seldom entirely ego syntonic, or conflict free. The therapist who takes the threat of violence seriously and discusses a proposed course of action with the patient, demonstrates an alliance with the healthier aspects of the patient's personality. When the therapist discusses a warning, he or she demonstrates the ability to remain concerned even in the face of imminent danger. In most cases, this strengthens the alliance. Consider what it would mean if the therapist stood passively by and permitted the patient to carry out the threat. The therapist's clinical responsibility to prevent his patient from harming another is at least as great as his responsibility to prevent the patient from harming him or herself. A legal duty to third persons exists when a patient threatens or acts violently, but the legal duty is secondary to the clinical duty to the patient. The clinical duty requires the therapist to explore the issue with the patient, and take whatever action seems appropriate under the circumstances (see below).

Stone has recently commented that the central ambiguity in *Tarasoff* is that it tells the psychotherapist that he or she must protect third parties, but does not specify what steps are legally necessary and sufficient to meet this obligation to protect the public (24). The foregoing argument implies that the ambiguity of *Tarasoff* is the ambiguity of clinical psychiatry. In the same way that we must decide what course of action to choose to best protect the patient, so we must decide what course to choose to best protect society. If we regard this as a therapeutic issue to be discussed with the patient, I believe that, in most cases, it will be possible to reach agreement with the patient on how best to proceed.

Once the clinician has made the assessment that a patient is potentially violent, the choice of action is limited, broadly speaking, to one of three: 1) Deal with the problem with the patient, within the therapy; 2) Discuss the problem with some third person, such as the victim and/or the police; 3) Hospitalize the patient, voluntarily if possible; or involuntarily if not, assuming the patient gives evidence of mental disorder sufficient to meet legal standards for involuntary commitment.

How should the clinician decide which course to follow? If he or she is satisfied, after discussing the matter thoroughly with the patient, that the patient will not be violent before the next scheduled appointment, then the clinician can afford to treat the potential violence as a purely therapeutic issue. If the therapist believes there is a real likelihood of serious violence within the next 24 to 48 hours, then hospitalization is the intervention of choice. In the most uncertain case, which is intermediate between the two, the clinician believes that violence is a distinct possibility, but does not believe it is imminent (such as Case Example One in Chapter Four). In this situation, discussing the problem with some third person, such as the victim, is usually the best choice. The clinician should consider Wechsler's (25) suggestion to involve the patient and the victim in conjoint discussions. Many clinicians are initially put off by this suggestion, but on reflection some have found it to be worthwhile.

Recent Court decisions limiting the *Tarasoff* duty to cases in which there is an identified victim decrease the ambiguity of the therapist's choice of action. For the broad middle range of potentially violent patients who are not committable, but who may be violent before the next session, warning seems to be the intervention of choice. Certainly, there is less ambiguity in dealing with a patient who threatens an individual, than in dealing with a patient like the "notorious masturbator" who threatened to firebomb a university (26).

Whenever the clinician is doubtful about an assessment of potential violence or about a course of action, he or she should discuss the problem with a valued colleague or supervisor. The clinician should also always write a careful note documenting the procedure used to assess violence; that is, specific questions asked and specific answers given. The note should contain the clinician's conclusion about the likelihood of violence, citing clinical data, a statement of what the clinician proposes to do, and the reasons why he or she believes the proposed choice will be effective. The consultant's opinion should also be recorded. If the clinician does all this, even if his or her judgment is wrong, and serious violence occurs, it is unlikely that a Court will find that the clinician has breached any legal duty.

RECOMMENDATIONS FOR THE FUTURE

A consensus appears to be emerging that the *Tarasoff* duty, as it relates to outpatients, should be limited to cases in which the patient has threatened or acted against a specific, identifiable victim. This is a sound rule.

For the potentially dangerous inpatient, I have suggested that the *Tarasoff* duty seldom provides additional safeguards for the public beyond those provided by current standards governing decisions to release. In most cases, the duty to use reasonable care according to a professional standard suffices to safeguard a foreseeable victim as well as the general public. Only if a patient is determined not to meet commitment standards, but is still thought to be potentially dangerous at the point of release, should a *Tarasoff* duty be invoked. In this case, the duty should also be specifically limited to cases in which the patient has threatened or acted against a specific identifiable victim.

Appelbaum's proposals for evaluating whether the psychotherapist has met the *Tarasoff* duty appear sound, and are worth repeating here. There is a professional standard for assessment of violence (26), and psychotherapists should be held to it.

There is no professional standard for prediction of violence. As argued in Chapter Five, the most we can expect of predictions is that they are accurate for a sample, but not necessarily in the individual case. Thus, psychiatrists and other psychotherapists should continue to predict violence, but the Courts should consider the predictions themselves to be negligent only if they are based on negligent assessment practices, or if they appear to show a reckless disregard for the facts.

When the therapist acts to meet the *Tarasoff* duty, the actions should be judged under a professional standard of negligence, not an ordinary standard. This means that the therapist's conduct is judged against the standard of what is good practice within the profession. When an ordinary standard is applied, as it was in *Tarasoff*, the standard is what a reasonable person would have done under the circumstances. Under a professional standard, other psychotherapists can render an expert opinion on whether the behavior met professional standards. Under ordinary negligence standards, the jury uses its own judgment of what a reasonable person would do. Since it is clear from many subsequent decisions that the *Tarasoff* duty rests on a special relationship that devolves because of the professional relationship between the psychotherapist and the patient, it seems reasonable to apply a professional standard in evaluating the adequacy of the therapist's actions. A similar argument applies for judging whether the psychotherapist has taken adequate steps to insure that the proposed course of action has been carried out.

References

1. The Principles of Medical Ethics, With Annotations Especially Applicable to Psychiatry. Washington, D.C., American Psychiatric Association, 1981

2. *Tarasoff v. Regents of the University of California*, 17 Cal. 3d 425, 551 P.2d 334 (1976)

3. *Tarasoff v. Regents of the University of California*, 118 Cal. Rptr. 129, 529 P.2d 553 (1974)

4. Deukmejian G: Letter to members of California Assembly, Governor's Office, Sacramento, September 28, 1984

5. *Hedlund v. Orange County*, 669 P.2d 41 (Cal. 1983)

6. *Jablonski v. U.S.*, 712 F.2d 391 (9th Cir. 1983)

7. *Thompson v. County of Alameda*, 167 Cal. Rptr. 70 (1980)

8. *McIntosh v. Milano*, 403 A.2d 500 (N.J. Supr. Ct. 1979)

9. *Peck v. Counseling Service of Addison County, Inc., Vt.* Addison Sup Ct, No. S114-80Ac (January 17, 1983)

10. *Shaw v. Glickman*, Md. App., 415A.2d 625, (1980)

11. *Brady v. Hopper*, 570 F. Supp. 1333 (D. Colo. 1983)

12. *Hopewell v. Adibempe*, No. GD78–28756, Civil Division, Court of Common Pleas of Allegheny County, Pennsylvania, June 1, 1981

13. *MacDonald v. Clinger*, App. Div., 446N.Y.S.2d 801 (1982)

14. *Davis v. Lhim*, Mich. Wayne County Circuit Court, No. 77-726989 NM (June 11, 1981)

15. *Petersen v. Washington*, 671 P.2d 230 (Wash. 1980)

16. *Chrite v. U.S.*, 564 F. Supp. 341, (1983)

17. *Furr v. Spring Grove State Hospital*, 53 Md. App.474, 454 A2d 414 (1983)

18. *Leedy v. Hartnett*, 519 F. Supp. 1125 (1981)

19. *Hasenei v. U.S.*, 541 F. Supp. 999 (D. Md. 1982)

20. *Holmes v. Wampler*, 546 F. Supp. 500 (EO VA 111982)

21. *Doyle v. U.S.*, 530 F. Supp. 1278 (C.D. Cal. 1982)

22. *Lipari v. Sears, Roebuck & Co.*, 497 F. Supp. 185 (D. Neb. 1980)

23. Wise TP: Where the public peril begins: a survey of psychotherapists to determine the effects of *Tarasoff*. Stanford Law Review 31:165–190, 1978

24. Stone AA: Law, Psychiatry, and Morality. Washington, D.C., American Psychiatric Press, 1984

25. Wechsler DB: Patients, therapists and third parties: the victimological virtues of *Tarasoff*. International Journal of Law and Psychiatry 2:1–28, 1979

26. Kroll J, Mackenzie TB: When psychiatrists are liable: risk management and violent patients. Hosp Community Psychiatry 34:29–37, 1983